MINI-MASSAGE

Other books by Jack Hofer

Total Massage

Stress Busters

Live Longer Now
(with Jon Leonard and Nathan Pritikin)

MINI-MASSAGE

JACK HOFER

Illustrations by
Dana Campbell

A Perigee Book

To Gretchen

Perigee Books
are published by
The Putnam Publishing Group
200 Madison Avenue
New York, NY 10016

Library of Congress Cataloging-in-Publication Data

Hofer, Jack L.
Mini-massage.

Includes index.
1. Massage. I. Title.
RM721.H55 1988 615.8'22 88-5830
ISBN 0-399-51468-6

Typeset by Fisher Composition, Inc.
Printed in the United States of America
1 2 3 4 5 6 7 8 9 10

CONTENTS

HOW TO USE THIS BOOK

Remember when you were little and in pain, and your mother or father would ask "Where does it hurt?" You would tell them, and they could help. Now, over the years, through the wear and tear of everyday life, you have probably found it less easy to locate and heal the pain. Each of us has areas that give us trouble from time to time. Maybe it's your lower back that goes out at the worst moment, or a kinked neck after a busy day on the phone, or a muscle spasm in your calf after an overly brisk jog. Even tiny muscles in our faces reflect tension and stress. In *Mini-Massage,* you will learn how to relieve specific muscle trouble spots with a simple, relaxing 10-15 minute mini-massage.

Many people don't realize how tense certain muscles are until they've had a good massage. For those who have never had a massage of any kind, a mini-massage is an easy way to start. It doesn't take a lot of time, and for the shy beginner, many of the movements can be done without removing any clothing. In fact, none of the movements require complete nudity.

You don't have to be hurting to benefit from a mini-massage. Though it is an excellent means of relieving muscle tension, it also feels great anytime. Mini-massage can improve performance in sports, business, and at home. Have one before or after an important event, as an energy pick-me-up, or as a way to relax in the evening. One of the benefits of a relaxed mind and body is an increase in your ability to withstand adverse stress. Frequent mini-massages also serve as a kind of preventive medicine. They enhance circulation and the ability of the immune system to do its job while reducing tension, nerve interference, and the output of excess adrenaline.

Mini-Massage breaks the parts of the body down and treats each part with different massage techniques. Beginning with a discussion of the increasing amount of stress and tension that affects all our lives, we proceed to a close look at the various parts of the body and how they react to stress. People suffering from pain in the head, face and neck may have direct muscle tension to be released, but may also be suffering from *referred pain*, that is, soreness or tenderness passed along the nerves from another part of the body. For instance, a number of back muscles tie into the tendons attached to the point where the neck joins the head. Tenderness is common in this spot.

Many people, office workers in particular, suffer from muscle tightness and pain in the shoulders and upper back. Sitting at a desk hunched over a phone, word processor or typewriter can contort this intricate series of muscles, and a mini-massage can provide fast relief.

Experts say that one out of every two people will experience mild to severe lower back pain at some time during his or her life. Along with simple mini-massages for this problem area, we provide techniques to strengthen and balance the lower back muscles.

Mini-massage can also help treat the internal tension that can make the abdomen a welter of problems. Ulcers, acid stomach, indigestion, constipation, diarrhea and colitis are all manifestations of tension. Certain massage movements can reduce the intestinal imbalance and help restore an orderly flow of digestion.

The Chinese have claimed for thousands of years that the feet are a focal point for bodily ills and well being. Certainly our legs and feet take a beating on all the concrete and asphalt of modern streets. A good foot and leg mini-massage can dissipate aches and pains magically.

If for some reason you don't have a partner handy to exchange massages with, don't worry. Detailed instructions for self-massage are given in Chapter 8, along with advice on using the variety of sophisticated massage accessories available today.

Mini-massage is not the only way to relieve stress and tension. Close self-surveillance can reveal a variety of anxiety and stress producers, from rapid, shallow breathing, or obsessive ceaseless concentration on one thing, to claustrophobia in traffic jams, or chronic impatience. You can do something about these patterns before you reach the breaking point. *Mini-Massage* offers exciting and varied ways to counteract daily stresses.

Finally, on a light note (since play is in itself an important stress buster), in Chapter 9 you'll find the results of a long-term survey of people who reached their one-hundredth birthday and a list of the main reason each gave for his or her long life. The pure contrariness of people will amaze and amuse you.

1

FAST-ACTION TENSION

As the pace of life quickens each year, more and more burdens seem to pile up. Houses, mortgages, taxes, insurance, international crises, anxieties over arms control or the trade deficit, and the sheer agony of getting to work in traffic every morning are just some of the factors contributing to the physical and mental stress of everyday life.

The remaining years before the twenty-first century will usher in technical and social changes more radical than those of any previous period in recent history. We, by nature, have a built-in anxiety about, and reluctance to, change. Super fast-paced change carries with it a taxing level of fast-action tension, and we'll need quick, foolproof ways to relieve it.

Massage has come of age. It's moved from massage studios into corporations, private offices, shopping centers, and most importantly, into the home. No longer is a home massage the luxury of a privileged few. Licensed massage therapists are making more and more out-of-studio visits to give mini-massages.

A mini-massage meets the needs of people in a fast-paced business world by helping them to relax and feel better. Their tight office and home schedules make a quick tune-up a more viable remedy for stress than the longer full-body massage. If you don't have the time or money for a full workup, a mini-massage is the perfect solution. It costs far less if given by a friend, spouse or family member.

People in all walks of life are discovering the benefits of a tune-up massage. A top lawyer in Seattle has one before each of his big court cases. An ad agency executive in Florida gets a massage twice a week—in her home. Her husband and daughter enjoy massages as well. A tax accountant in Massachusetts regularly gets a shoulder and back massage from one of the members of his family. He requires one almost every day during the first quarter of the year, when requests for help and preparation of income tax returns pour in.

A writer in Colorado schedules a facial massage and work on his neck and shoulders every Friday afternoon. He finds a mini-massage is an excellent way to end the work week and relax and refocus him for a day or two away from the writing routine. These days, he gets three mini-massages for the cost of a single full-body massage. When time and money permit, he still gets a complete body massage, but he finds the short version is well suited to his tight schedule.

Nurses use daily mini-massages to soothe hospital patients. They may call it a backrub, but the purpose, like that of a mini-massage, is to help the patient relax, to relieve his or her fears and reduce pain, and to help the patient sleep. Two nurses in Oregon who live in the same building trade off giving each other a mini-massage. When one nurse returns from her shift, especially if it's been a rough night, she goes to the other nurse for a 10 minute mini-massage before she, in turn, leaves for her shift.

A high-flying commodity floor trader in Chicago says he keeps a regular appointment with a massage therapist to "help keep his head on straight." He schedules a mini-massage every afternoon if he's taking big hits in the market—it makes no difference whether he's winning or losing. He says, "I'll give up some of my luxuries, but I won't give up my mini-massages."

An English rock superstar gets a shoulder and back rubdown before each concert. Bob Hope has a full-time massage therapist who travels with him and gives special body work as necessary. In Denver, there are massage therapists who spend a whole day at a single company giving 15 minute mini-massages to each of the employees. Now that's a company benefit.

Olympic and professional athletes routinely get therapeutic mini-massages to relax sore, tight muscles and to help prevent muscle spasms. Mini-massage also aids in recovery from many sports-related injuries.

PREVENTIVE HEALTH CARE

A mini-massage helps keep your stress level in a safe range. Your personal stress level is just the amount of stress you're under at any given time. To help visualize your stress level, let's imagine that the total scale from a relaxed, mellow state to a nervous breakdown is 3 feet long. If your normal stress level is about one-third of the way down the scale, you are a safe distance from total system overload.

However, if you are living only 3 inches from the breakdown point, it won't take much to push you into a crisis. You may know of someone who went over the edge, or even died, after some seemingly small thing triggered a massive, wild reaction.

Massages, chiropractic and osteopathic care are some of the ways of giving general body tune-ups. The goal of all preventive health care, regardless of what form it may take, is to keep your body working at its best. Other means of keeping the body running smoothly include nutrition, exercise, sports, and simply enjoying your life and your work.

But you don't have to live a few inches away from your critical stress point. Frequent mini-massages help build up your stress endurance. By relaxing your muscles and stimulating your nerve ends, they help your nerves carry soothing, reassuring physical messages back and forth from your brain, through the spinal cord, to the muscles, organs and the rest of your body. If you are close to your critical stress point, chiropractic or osteopathic care can be used along with mini-massages. These types of health care focus on correcting interference and blockage in the nervous system so that the body can perform at its best. Along with manipulation to effect spinal adjustments, chiropractors and osteopaths relax the muscles, using devices such as diathermy machines, muscle stimulators, heavy-duty vibrators, and vibrating tables. Easing blockages of nerve energy helps your body go about its daily business without excess pain and strain.

Though it is important to keep the body working at peak performance, it is equally necessary to be able to relax during and at the end of the day. Some people find that hobbies, sports, exercise, TV, movies, theater, eating out, working in the yard, visiting friends and other things are a means of letting go. Everyone has a certain activity (or nonactivity) that makes them feel relaxed and at ease. You have to discover what it is that helps you to relax and unwind.

Negative emotions and muscle tension go together. A study at the National Heart and Lung Institute showed that being angry, impatient and highly competitive, even in small matters, puts a person at a higher risk of a heart attack or stroke. A study of 670 mid- and upper-level managers at a utility company in Illinois showed that those who were open to challenge and change felt more in control of their lives, and had far less illness requiring sick leave during the year. In another medical study at the Stanford Research Institute it was found that the emotion most likely to lead to sudden death is *anger*.

Blood and hormonal research shows that your serum cholesterol goes up during a period of acute stress. When you are shocked, or put instantly on the defensive, your brain produces ACTH (adrenocorticotropic hormone), which jolts your adrenal glands to produce adrenaline. Some doctors feel that repeated or long-term episodes of excess adrenaline production due to negative stress can cause the muscles of the heart to weaken and work unevenly, which, in turn, heightens your chance of having a heart attack.

For years Paul Harvey, the Chicago newscaster, has talked about the link between severe stress and serious illness. It is one of those things that many people feel affect our life and health. However, stress isn't an easy variable to single out in controlled medical studies, so its actual role in illness stirs up a lot of controversy.

FREQUENT MINI-MASSAGES

Frequent mini-massages help you maintain your stress level within a safe range. A mini-massage works directly on spots of acute muscle tension and helps you to relax and let go. This in turn aids your circulatory and neural systems in doing their jobs, while your body produces fewer harmful chemicals and rids itself of toxins more easily.

I haven't provided any anatomical, acupuncture, acupressure, meridian, foot/hand reflexology, chakra or other charts in this book. These healing disciplines are just a few of the many ways we have learned over the ages to counteract stress and restore physical and mental harmony. The movement of energy around and through the hundreds of miles of neural pathways throughout the body is dealt with by keeping the connections clear so the nerve impulses can do what they're supposed to do. Mini-massage helps keep these pathways and connections clear and open.

2

TARGET STRESS AREAS

A mini-massage doesn't mean a fast or hurried massage. It means focusing your attention completely for 10-15 minutes on one or two areas of the receiver's body. Don't even try to give a mini-massage if you can't spend at least 10 minutes without interruptions. Anything less just isn't enough time to work the tension out of tight muscles.

Certain jobs seem to make for tension in specific muscles. Barbers, beauticians, salesclerks, restaurant workers and others who spend the work day walking and standing on hard floors often have trouble with cramps in their legs and feet. Secretaries, writers, editors, computer operators, programmers, typists and others working at a keyboard or desk register tension in their upper back, shoulders and neck. Truck drivers and people doing a lot of lifting often have problems in their lower back.

You need two or more muscles to keep any part of your body erect or to move an arm, hand, finger, leg, foot or your head. One set of muscles contracts to move your arm in one direction and a different muscle contracts to reverse direction. Sitting at a desk all day with your shoulders hunched puts constant strain on certain muscles in the shoulders and back, which, over a period of time raises the threshold of muscle tension to higher and higher levels. When this goes on year after year, muscles can assume a fixed, unnatural shape or condition, occasionally becoming so hard that they ossify (form bony matter).

Muscle tension this ingrained needs repeated treatments in order to break the rigid habit and allow the muscles to relax once again.

That part of your nervous system which gives you the energy to run or fight, triggers the secretion of adrenaline, which is hard to turn off once it's turned on. Adrenaline also lowers the threshold necessary for the nerves to fire and causes the muscles to be at "red alert." This is why a person on the verge of a nervous breakdown is sometimes jumpy and easily startled by normal sounds. Since our bodies are largely made up of muscle tissue, and muscles contract under stress, stress-related illnesses always show their signs, however faintly, somewhere in the muscles.

When your body is suddenly aroused by some event, specific muscles contract or "clamp down" and your heart rate and blood pressure go up. If the arousal is long-term, you may feel like you're in a vise from the pressure in your tense muscles.

Repeated muscle tension in a given area can cause semipermanent changes in your body posture unless something is done to break the cycle. If you hold any position for a long enough time, your muscles will tend to keep you in that position. Certain muscles end up doing all the work while others do practically nothing. Instead of a balanced lengthening and shortening, one group becomes shorter and tenses as the other group lengthens and relaxes. After a while, this imbalance reflects itself as pain in the muscles and may cause your body to reshape itself or even cause vertebrae in the spine to rotate or move out of place.

People with rounded shoulders, a hump in their backs, head pushed forward or body leaning to the right or left generally have certain muscles in a fixed state of contraction, keeping them in that position. Also, many common headaches result from tense muscles in the face, neck and shoulders. With practice it's easy for a person to locate muscles under tension by sensing a muscle's "tightness." This is especially noticeable when you feel tension in the back and upper shoulders. You can place your hand on these areas and actually feel that the muscles are hard and tight. A mini-massage will help your body assume a more natural, relaxed posture.

Another type of muscle trouble is the spasm, or charley horse.

This occurs when certain muscles lock into a repeated series of contractions. Usually the source of the trouble is a deep, localized spot of intense pain called a trigger point. It may even feel hot around the area.

Certain disorders result from a group of tense muscles in target areas such as the back, shoulders or neck; certain types of diarrhea or constipation in the digestive system, for example. These tense muscles refer their pain along nerve circuits to the head and jaw, among other sites of the body. This locked or frozen energy has no place to go. Once you relieve the tense muscles, the frozen energy releases from the referred-pain sites, and an orderly flow restores the target area to its normal resting state.

Muscle stress or tension manifests itself in varying ways. Some people bite their nails, hunch their shoulders, grind their teeth or clench their jaws. Others wring their hands, wrap one leg tightly around the other, fold their arms tightly across their chests, or drum their fingers on the desk. Still others tap their feet, wiggle around in their chairs, emit nervous laughs, jump at the slightest sound, or frown a lot. Check yourself for nervous symptoms and develop mini-massages especially for the affected areas.

ADVANTAGES OF A MINI-MASSAGE

The main advantage of a mini-massage is that it only takes 10–15 minutes to give or receive one. A harried homemaker in Washington state says, "A mini-massage is the best 10 minutes of my day. My husband knows how much it relaxes me. Even the older children get into the act of working on me."

Another advantage of a mini-massage is that it doesn't wear out the giver. Two people can easily give each other a mini-massage the same day, although it's nice to switch the order of who receives the last massage.

You may give or receive a mini-massage almost anywhere you

can find privacy—at home, in the office, or when traveling. It's important however to find a place where you won't be disturbed for at least 15 minutes. If you're at work, you can go into an office. Post a Do Not Disturb sign on the door. Anyone who has had a massage knows that it's important not to be interrupted while it's in progress.

While traveling, one of the passengers can give the driver a 10 minute mini-massage of the shoulders and upper back at the end of the day's drive. If you're traveling alone and feel you need some massage work, check at the desk of the hotel or motel you're staying in and ask if they can recommend a good massage therapist. Many massage therapists have portable tables or portable massage chairs and are often willing to make out-of-office calls during the evening. Or if it's during normal business hours, you can go to their office.

If you're at home, make sure you're not disturbed during the session. Evening is a good time for massaging people who have trouble sleeping or who have something pressing on their minds. Mini-massages at home are also good during times of crisis or during lean economic times, when spending money is tight. They are certainly more relaxing than many of today's movies.

Studies show massage helps active people in several ways. It causes the blood vessels to dilate, increases the rate of exchange of substances in the blood, and it decreases pulse rate while raising muscle efficiency. Massage reduces lactic acid levels in muscle, reduces swelling and helps prevent excessive scar tissue from forming in torn muscles. It also helps retain nitrogen, phosphorus and sulfur needed for healing broken bones.

TARGET AREAS OF TENSION

People who ask for a massage often have a specific part of their body that they want worked on. So instead of having a total massage, they often prefer an intense mini-massage on the one or two most tense areas.

One person may enjoy a soothing foot and calf massage, while another finds relief in a massage of their lower back. Some like combined work done on more than one part of the body such as face and upper back, or midsection and lower back. You can even spend 10–15 minutes just giving full-length strokes on the front and/or back of a person's body. Couples can give each other short mini-massages on a daily basis.

Athletes and people who work out suffer pain from two causes: overuse and injury. The better the shape you're in, the less likely you are to suffer injury or pain from overuse. The key element is to build up strength and endurance in a gradual way and to use massage when necessary to relieve soreness in your muscles. A mini-massage can even improve your performance. If pain or injury does occur you may compensate by limping or holding the injured area in a set position. As mentioned before, this can change your posture and physical balance. A gentle mini-massage of the injured area helps restore use and normal posture. Professional athletes say that recovery is faster and less painful with the use of massage.

Early in 1987, the boxer "Sugar Ray" Leonard trained for 2½ months at the Hotel Inter-Continental for his upcoming fight with "Marvelous" Marvin Hagler. Early in training, Sugar Ray had complained of a pinched nerve in his neck, and although several neurosurgeons had urged him to take prescribed drugs, he absolutely refused.

He learned of Henry Wingfield, the massage therapist at the hotel's health club, and decided to try a mini-massage. After his first mini-massage Sugar Ray sat up and said in astonishment, "My God, I've never felt like this before . . . and I'm not dizzy. You fixed it!"

Henry continued to give Sugar Ray 15 minute mini-massages during the cool-down period after each daily workout. Even the trainers and others in his support staff wound up getting mini-massages. Sugar Ray went on to win the fight.

At Stockholm's Karolinska Institute, Swedish exercise physiologist Nina Ask studied the strength and endurance of eight cyclists.

After one series of repeated high-intensity workouts, they rested for 10 minutes. Then she tested them for strength and endurance. After repeating the same series of workouts, each received 10 minutes of massage. She again tested them for strength and endurance, and their performance rose by 11 percent. Ask credits the positive results to the reduction of lactic acid in the muscles, which was brought about by massage. Also, she says that muscles relax because of the sense of overall well-being one gets from a massage. She thinks massage between matches can improve the performance of tennis players. Track and field contestants also benefit from massages given between events. J. Meagher and P. Boughton, in their book, *Sportsmassage,* point out that cross-fiber massage and pressure on trigger points improve performance and endurance, and add to the athlete's "lifetime."

SOOTHING/HEALING ENERGY

The ancient Hawaiian *kahuna*s, or healers, used a powerful form of healing massage to treat a variety of injuries, from cuts and bruises to broken bones. It's reported by Hawaiian descendants that the kahunas employed a high form of fusion energy in which they massaged the injured part while picturing the injury as already being healed. They reportedly accomplished healing in less than 30 minutes that would normally take days, weeks or even months. Although it's not the purpose of this book to teach this form of healing—it usually takes years to reach such an advanced state—it's possible for you to send a limited form of soothing and balancing energy to the person receiving a mini-massage. In *Mini-Massage*, this form of energy transfer is mainly used to reduce muscle tension.

Although the kind of "instant" healing used by the kahunas is rare, people regularly use a limited form of hands-on healing. Mothers and fathers rub or kiss a child to take away the "hurt." Nurses have been using a form of therapeutic touch for many years to relieve hospital patients' pain.

In the movie *The Karate Kid*, Ralph Macchio—Daniel—experiences a form of quick healing. After agreeing to learn karate from an older friend, Pat Morita—Miyagi—in order to defend himself from a school bully, Daniel agrees to do whatever Miyagi requires of him. Daniel spends the next several days waxing Miyagi's collection of classic cars, sanding a huge outdoor deck and painting both sides of several hundred feet of fence surrounding Miyagi's home. All the time, Daniel keeps thinking to himself that this meaningless work has little or nothing to do with mastering the art of karate.

Unknown to Daniel, Miyagi is using these work projects to build up Daniel's hand and arm strength and the speed of his reflexes. By the end of the third day of ceaseless work, Daniel's shoulder is killing him, and he's about ready to quit for good when Miyagi rubs his hands together and places them on Daniel's shoulder. The pain disappears within a matter of seconds. He can't believe Miyagi healed him so quickly!

A certain amount of energy radiates out from your hands. You can warm the palms of your hands by briskly rubbing them together. When your hands are then laid on another's skin, this heat can be felt. As you give someone a mini-massage, think of your hands as two powerful heat lamps. See this warm energy pouring out from each hand into the muscles of the receiver. Nothing may happen at first, as it takes practice to learn to give out soothing energy. Keep envisioning this energy going out from your hands each time you give a mini-massage; the receiver will begin to notice a more and more relaxed feeling.

PREPARING FOR A MINI-MASSAGE

Even though it takes 10–15 minutes to give a mini-massage, you need to prepare the environment to make the person receiving the massage as comfortable as possible. The first thing to do is find a quiet place. It should be a room where you won't be disturbed for 15 minutes. Take the telephone off the hook so you won't be interrupted by calls in the middle of a massage. Music is OK if the person receiving the massage doesn't mind. Soft instrumental music can be relaxing. Remember to make the room warm enough. Even in the summer a person may get chilled when lying down since the body loses five times more heat in that position than when standing up. If necessary, cover the person with a blanket or sheet even though they are wearing clothing.

Almost as important as room temperature is the warmth of your hands. Cold hands can ruin the beginning of an otherwise good massage. It's like having someone sneak up behind you and drop an ice cube down the back of your shirt. If your hands are cold, rub them together briskly or run hot water over them until they are nice and warm.

Complete nudity isn't necessary when receiving a mini-massage, although there's nothing wrong with removing all clothing if the receiver feels comfortable. Obviously, clothing may be left on for a head, face and neck massage. It's optional for the upper back and shoulders. For work on the lower body, a person wearing a tight skirt may want to remove it to allow maximum access. Shorts may be worn for mini-massages of the legs, feet, lower back or stomach and midsection.

Before you start, ask the person to take five deep breaths. As you're giving the massage, remind her to keep breathing. You'll find people tend to hold their breath when you work on or near tender areas. This creates tension and fights against the soothing effects of the massage.

Long nails can be a hindrance so watch the length of your fingernails. Also make sure there aren't any sharp or jagged edges on your finger- or thumbnails. Unless instructed to do otherwise you will use the pads of your fingers and thumbs for most of the movements. See that your fingers flow evenly without jerky motions. Make the transition between movements as smooth as possible and maintain hands-on contact with the receiver as much as possible.

Mold your hands to fit the surface curves of the body part you're working on. Use even speed and pressure—don't rush any movement. (Pressure is indicated with each of the mini-massage movements as gentle, light, medium, firm or heavy.) Keep your hands, arms and shoulders relaxed as you do a mini-massage. Instead of using muscle power only, let the weight of your upper body provide leverage for the heavier movements, especially when you're massaging the back or shoulders. Leaning into the movements, while keeping your back as straight as possible, will help prevent fatigue in your shoulders and back. Don't worry about feeling clumsy or awkward, you'll pick up the right rhythm and speed quicker than you think.

If you've never given any kind of massage before, it's a good idea during the first few sessions to ask the person you're working on to tell you whether you're using too much or too little pressure. Remind them to let you know if you're causing any undue pain. A little pain is natural when working on sore muscles, but intense, throbbing pain could cause more overall tension than relief.

If you give or receive mini-massages often, you may want to buy or build your own massage table. Also available are the newer style massage chairs which are great for working on the neck, shoulders, arms and upper back. Massage tables and chairs are described in Chapter 8.

MASSAGE OILS AND CREAMS

Not all the mini-massage movements call for the use of oils. The best way to decide when to use a skin lubricant is to try doing each of the areas with and without one. Since massage has become so popular, a variety of massage oils, creams and lotions are now available at health stores and drugstores. Even some supermarkets carry these products in their health or cosmetics section. If you purchase a prepared product, look for one that's not heavily scented and one that contains more natural than artifical ingredients. I like to make up my own massage oil by adding a drop or two of a natural scent, such as wintergreen, clove or rose, to a natural coconut or almond oil.

If you use massage oil or cream, apply it only to the part of the body you are working on at the time. Don't try to cover the whole area at once. The skin will absorb the lubricant before you actually get to all the parts to be worked on, which is a waste of your oil or cream.

CHILDREN AND THE ELDERLY

Children's skin is smooth and pliant, and their muscles are supple and flexible. Mini-massage is great for children as their tense muscles repond easily to all the mini-massage movements, and they tend to relax more quickly than adults. Unfortunately, they aren't as likely to want to lie still for very long.

Special care should be taken when giving the elderly mini-massages. Although they like a soothing massage as much as younger people, their skin is thinner and tends to bruise more easily when too much pressure is used. When massaging an elderly friend or relative, use only gentle to medium pressure. Never use heavy pressure. And don't massage areas where bruises, wounds or varicose veins are present. It will only aggravate the problem. Older people also suffer from dry skin. You should use a moisturizing cream or oil each time you give them a massage.

3

HEAD, FACE AND NECK

TENSION IN HEAD, FACE AND NECK

The head, face and neck are prime areas for muscle tension. Whether you're in a good or a bad mood, your facial expressions serve as a mirror for your emotions. If you're down or in a bad mood, you're likely to have tension around the temples, the forehead and the mouth. Your neck is probably stiffer than normal, and the spot where your neck joins the back of your head is almost certain to feel tight and tender.

But mood is only one of many sources of tension and soreness in the face and neck. Your work habits and how you sit and stand during your waking hours can make you tense. A few simple changes of habit, and exercises, help to relieve this tension.

A booking agent in Michigan spends several hours a day on the phone and regularly complains of a sore neck. This problem is due to the bad habit of cradling the phone handset between the ear and upper shoulder, which places an undue strain on the neck. Even with a plastic shoulder cradle attachment for the handset, tension can build in the neck after frequent phone calls throughout the day.

If "hands-free" telephone conversation is necessary, it's better to use a high-quality speaker phone, which won't make your voice sound like you're in a cave or hollow barrel. Or, you can use an operator-type headset with microphone. If you must cradle the hand-set between your ear and shoulder or hold the handset to your ear in the normal way, you will be able to avoid excessive muscle soreness on one side of your neck by switching hands and sides throughout the day.

The jaw is a natural tension spot for people doing a lot of talking—salespeople, stock brokers and traders, insurance and travel agents, and teachers, for example. To relieve this tension, stop talking for a few moments—wiggle your jaw from side to side a few times, open your mouth as wide as possible, and then, let your jaw and tongue relax. Incessant gum chewing also can make your jaw hinge sore. The cure for tension caused by gum chewing is simple—spit out the gum.

There is a condition called TMJ (temporomandibular joint) dysfunction, which is a fancy name for certain problems with the jaw hinge and a person's bite. Many dentists believe an improper bite, or meshing of the teeth, to be responsible for putting an unnatural pressure on the temporal region of the skull. This pressure builds up and is a major source of many tension headaches. Experts suggest biting down hard on a 1–2 inch paperback for 10 seconds, then releasing it, as a way to relieve pain in the TMJ. This forces the jaw muscles to contract completely, then relax. It may be rough on the paperback, but if it helps, you can always chew on one you don't like.

The eyes are another common location for tension. If you've been doing a lot of reading, watching a computer screen, performing close handwork or driving, your eyes will tend to become tired and dry. I've described a simple, soothing technique to help relax tired eyes in Chapter 8.

HEAD, FACE AND NECK MOVEMENTS

The person receiving the mini-massage should be lying down on a massage table or on the floor. If you use the floor make sure it's carpeted, lay down some kind of padding—blanket, foam rubber pad, or a fully-inflated air mattress—to make the person comfortable. A bed works nicely as long as the person can lie down in a comfortable position with her head resting near the edge of the bed. The giver can sit on a chair near the edge of the bed, as long as all parts of the head and neck can be easily reached.

Use a light massage oil or cream to reduce friction and to help your fingers glide over the skin of the face. It feels wonderful, as well.

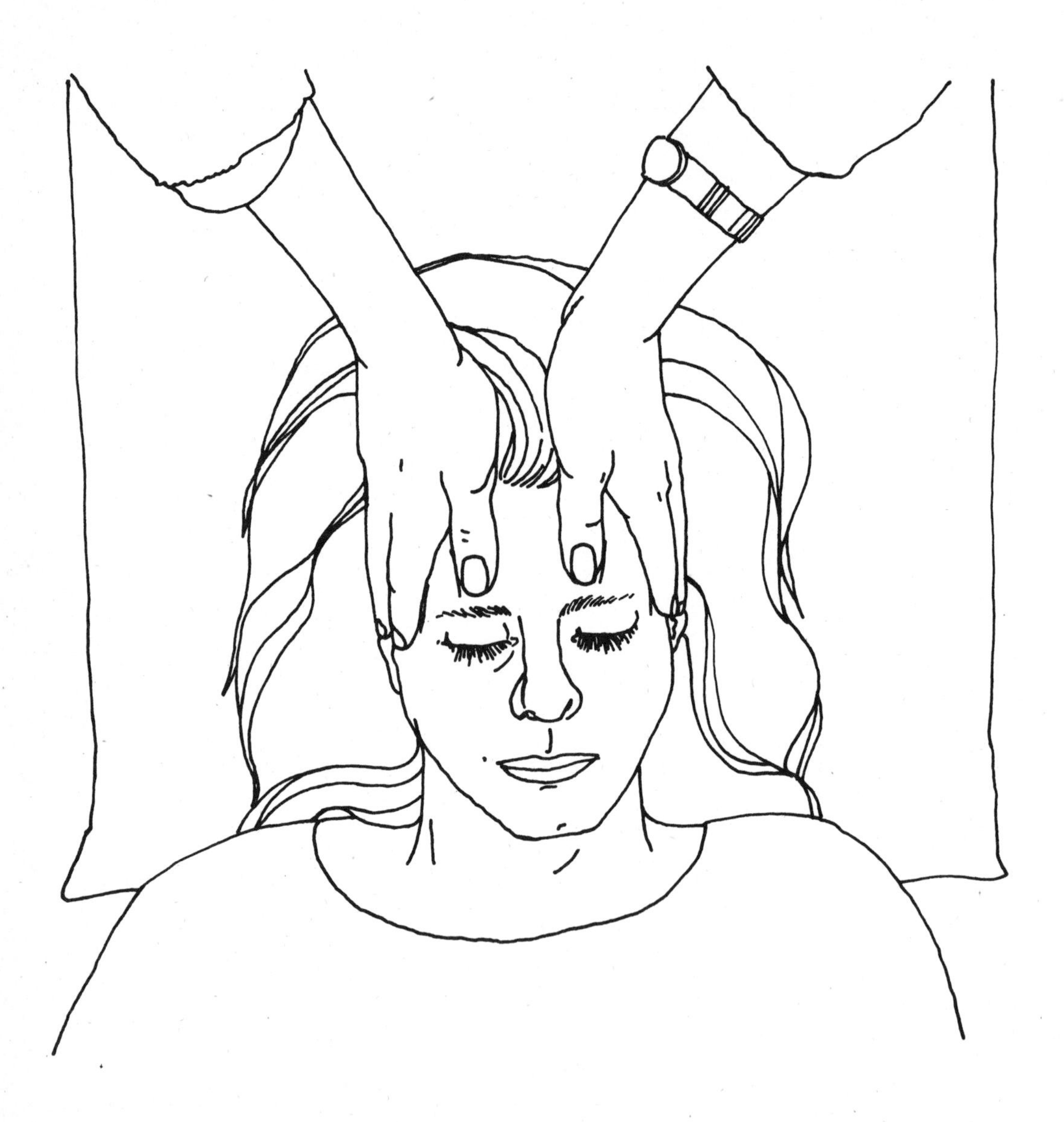

FOREHEAD

Start in the center of the forehead and use the thumb pads to iron out lines to the edge of the hairline.

Work in rows from just above the eyebrows up to the top of the forehead. Use light to medium pressure.

Another soothing movement is to use the pads of the first two or three fingers and make small circles all over the forehead.

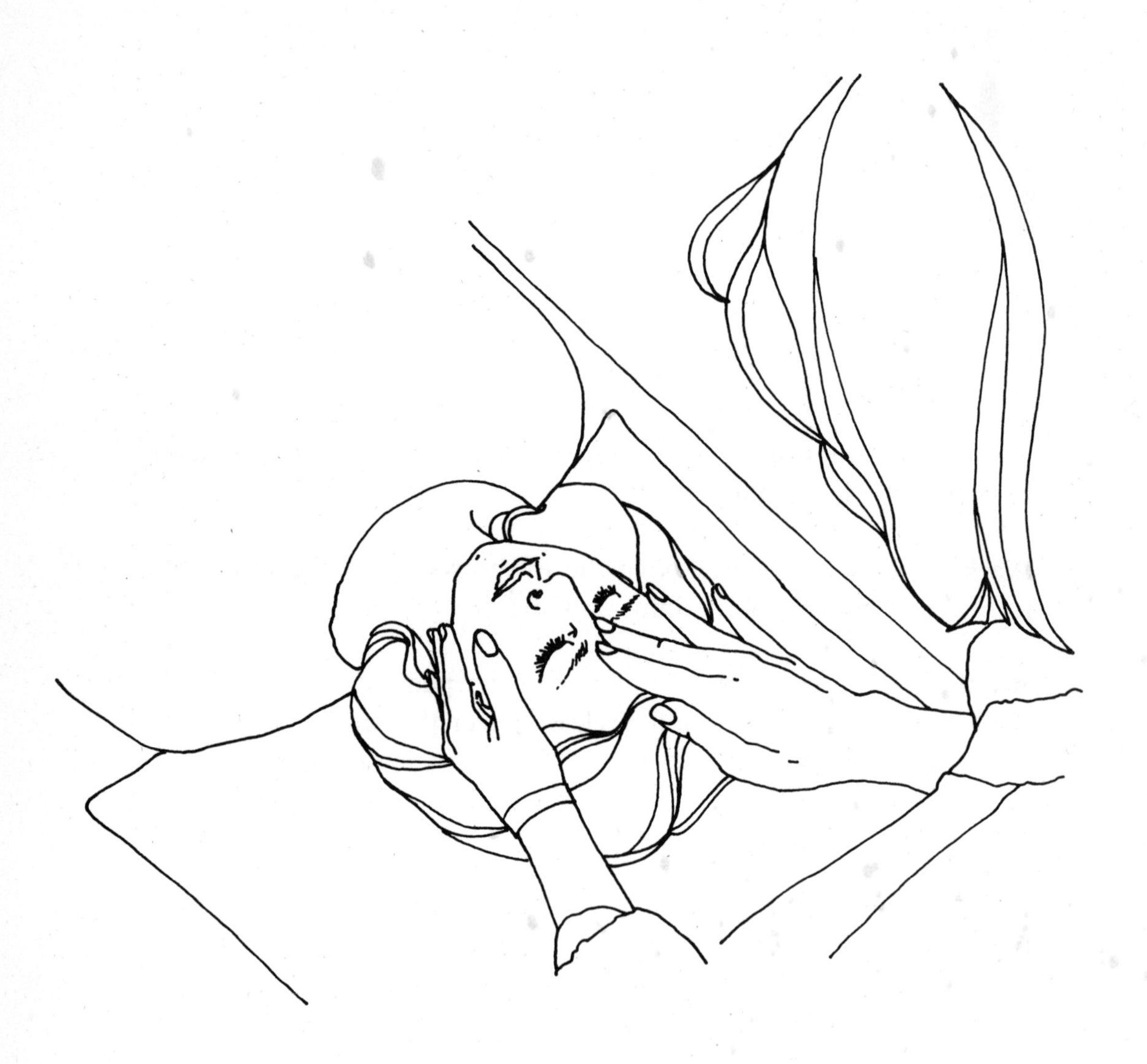

BETWEEN EYES

Use the pads of the first two fingers of one hand and stroke from the bridge of nose to top of the forehead.

If the person has furrows or deep lines in her forehead, spend extra time stroking and ironing out the skin. Use light to medium pressure.

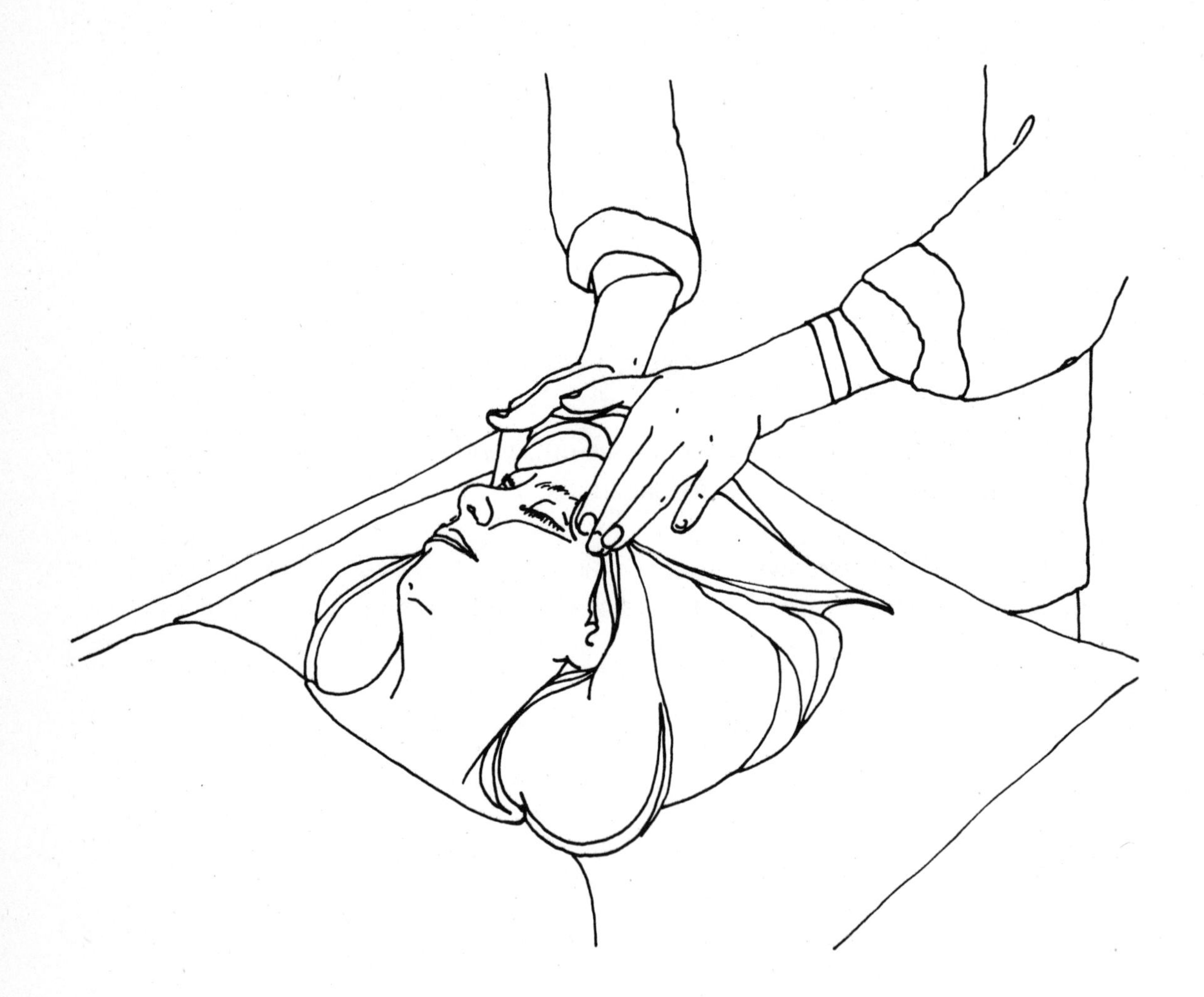

TEMPLES

Use the pads of the first two fingers of both hands to make tiny circles all around the temples. Use light to medium pressure.

Reverse circle direction several times.

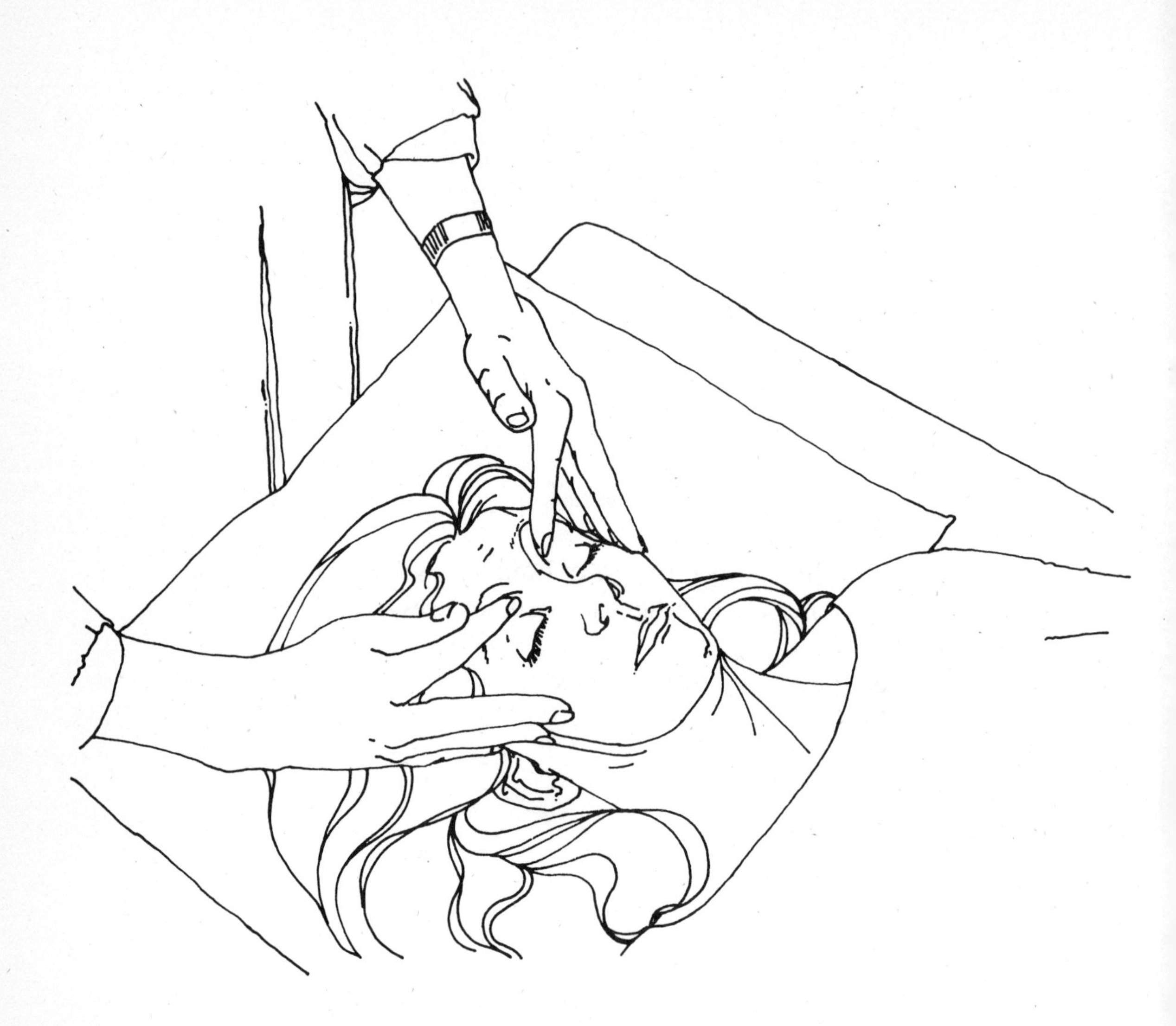

AROUND EYES

Carefully, with the forefingers or thumbs, stroke from the bridge of the nose along the upper eye socket ridge to the outside corner of the eyes. Do not put pressure on or poke the closed eyes.

Next stroke from the nose along the lower eye socket ridge to corner of eyes.

Go very slowly. Use light to medium pressure.

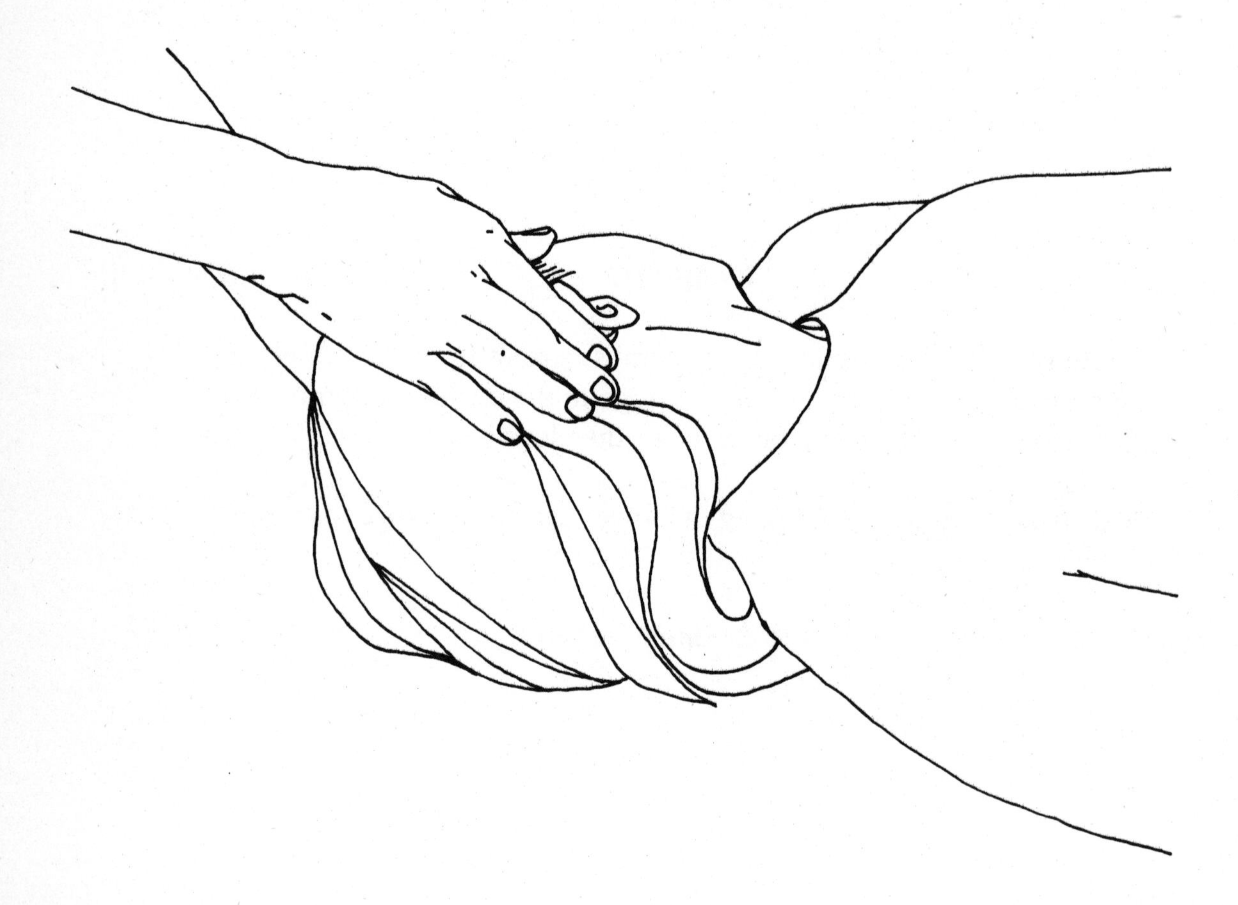

BEHIND EARS

Use the pads of the first two or three fingers of each hand to rub in small circles along the bone behind each ear, working from the bottom to the top and back to the bottom. Use medium to firm pressure.

As a change, stroke up and down along this bone. You can also gently stroke the ears themselves between your thumbs and the first two fingers. (Be sure to remove earrings.)

Use light pressure.

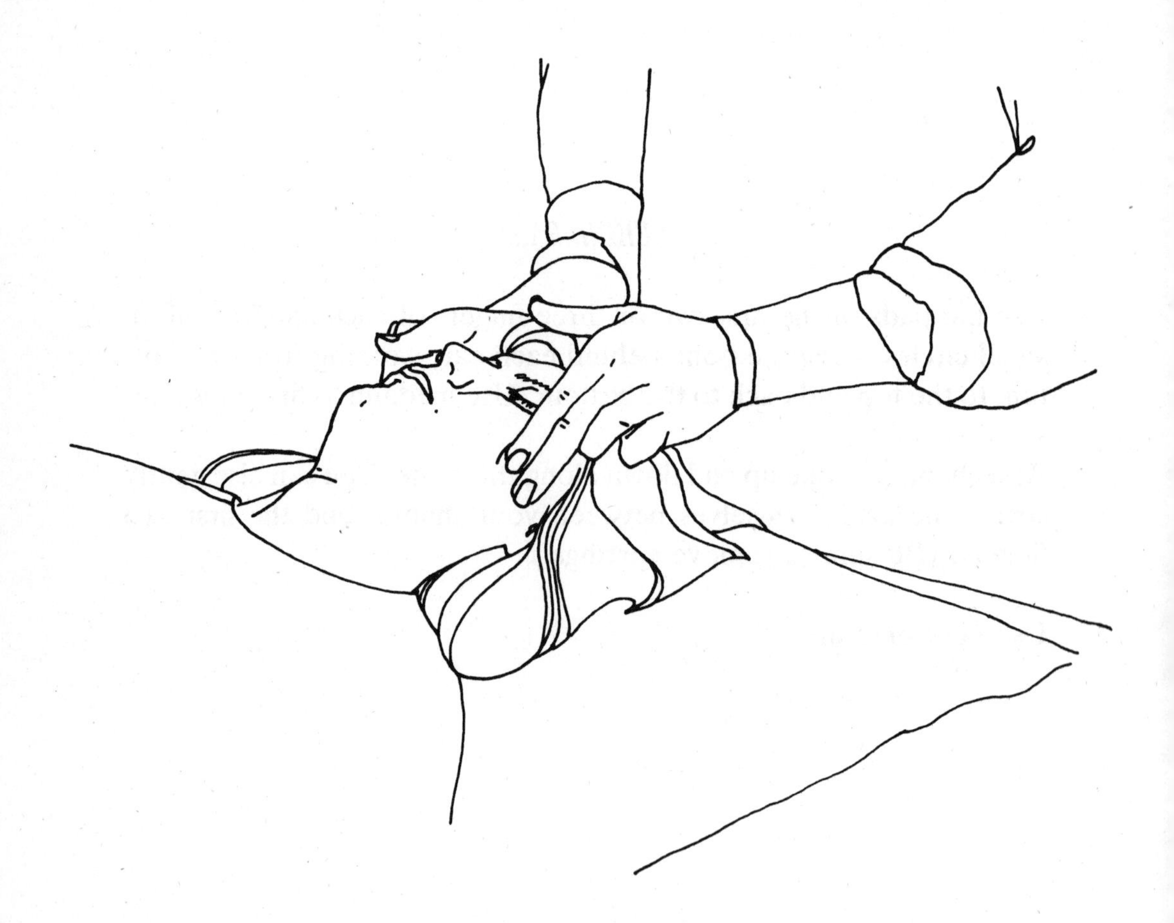

JAW

Use the pads of the first two fingers of each hand to make circles around the jaw hinge on the side of face. Follow along the lower jawbone to the base of the chin. Use medium pressure.

Reverse and go from base of the chin to upper jawbone.

As a variation, you can slowly stroke along the bottom of the jaw from the center where the jawbone angles up toward the ear. Make this a type of pulling stroke that moves the skin slightly over the jawbone as you work upward toward the ear from the base of the chin.

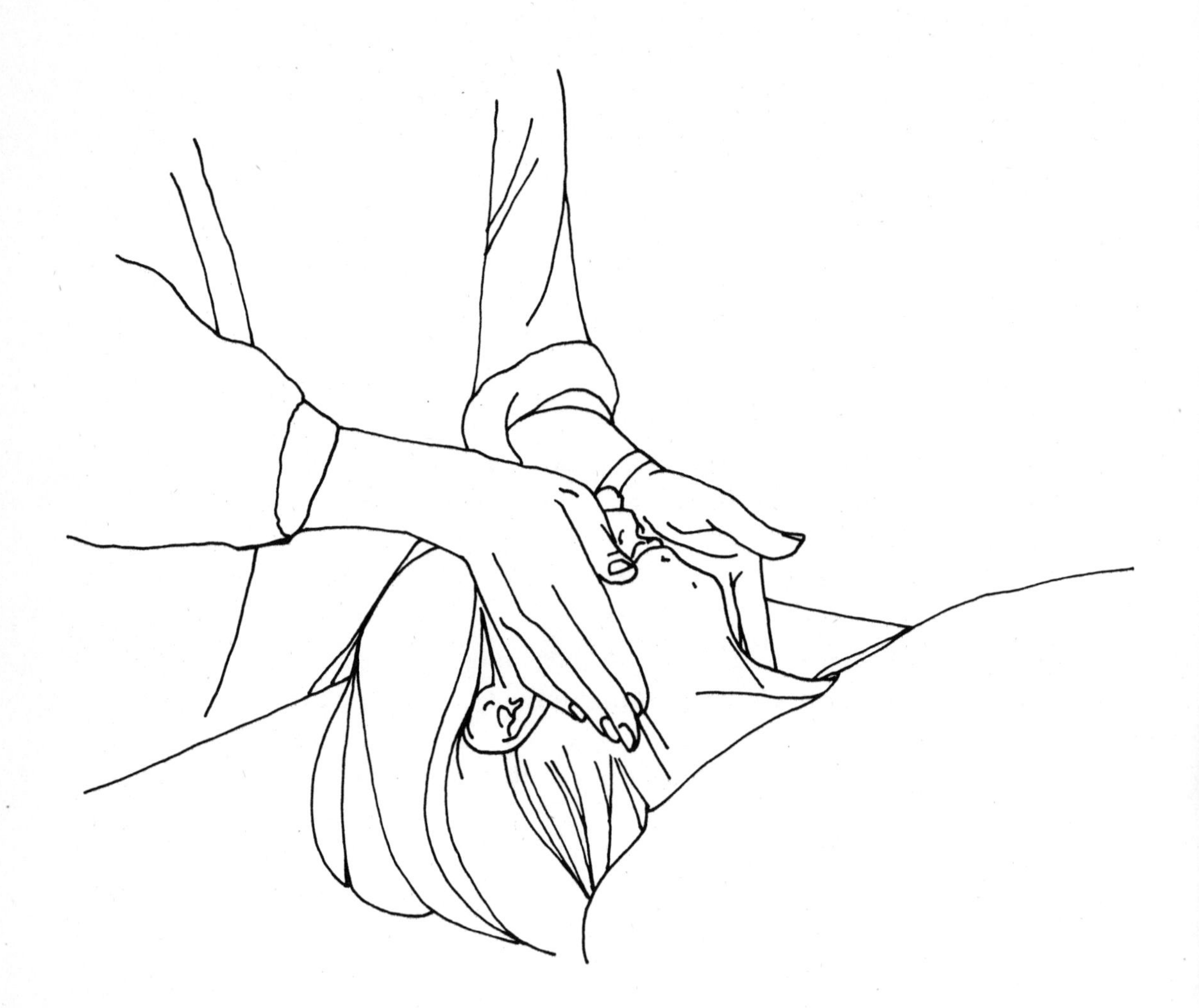

ALONG NECK

Use the pads of the first three fingers to make small circles along the neck. Work only on the sides and back of the neck. Do not massage around the windpipe.

Move from the upper ridge of the shoulders to the bone behind the ears and back again. Repeat several times. Use medium to firm pressure.

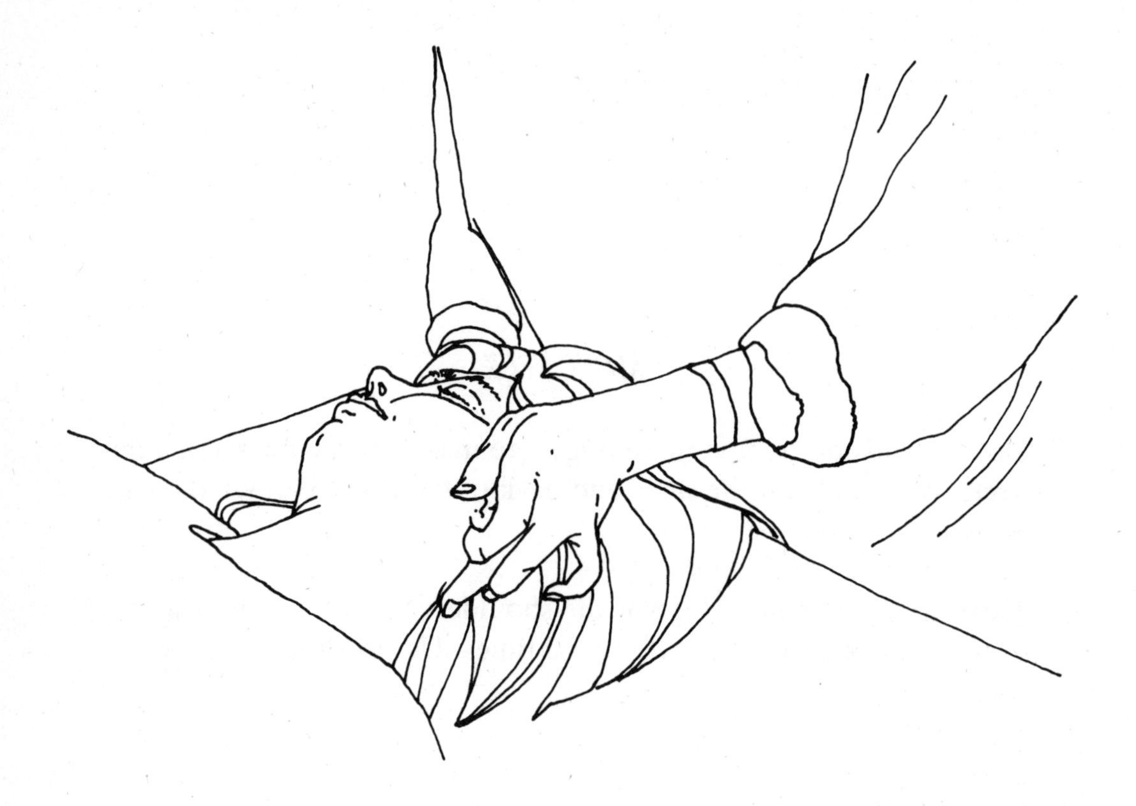

TREPIDATION

Use the pads of the first two fingers of each hand to apply firm, pulsing pressure at the point where the neck meets the lower back ridge of the skull.

Since this area is a major point of soreness for many people, keep the pulsing movement going for up to 3 minutes. Use firm pressure.

Instead of, or in addition to, using the pulsing movement, you can apply steady firm pressure for 10 seconds and then release for a few seconds and then repeat. Continue this sequence for up to 3 minutes.

Add a few light strokes to even out and relax the back of the neck after completing this pressure movement.

Keep repeating any of the movements for the entire 10–15 minutes. Some people like to have a lot of time spent working on their forehead and between the eyes. People who wear glasses like soothing movements on their temples. Those who habitually clench their teeth or talk a lot respond to work along the jaw. Ask the receiver what specific areas she wants you to work on.

FACIALS

Barbers, beauticians and hair stylists have been offering facials as part of their services for many years. You can add a pleasant touch to the above movements by using a few of their techniques.

After you finish the head, face and neck mini-massage, soak a couple of large cotton balls in cool water, squeeze out the excess water and place the balls over the closed eyelids. Next soak a towel in hot water, then twist the towel to remove the excess. If the towel is too hot, fan it in the air a few times to bring the temperature down. Place the warm towel around and over the face, covering all of the face except for the nose. Leave in place for 3–4 minutes.

Remove the towel and apply a light base of moisturizing cream if desired.

4

SHOULDERS AND UPPER BACK

TENSION IN SHOULDERS AND UPPER BACK

The shoulders and upper back are a familiar target area of muscle tension for office workers, especially those working long hours at typewriters, computers, word processors or other office machines. Part of the reason for this tension is improper working height of the machines. You need to be able to adjust the chair and desk so the machine is at a comfortable height. The keyboard should be at a height that allows your forearms to be bent slightly upward while letting your shoulders hang loosely. Ophthalmologists and optometrists say that when using a computer you should adjust the monitor screen to eye level. That way, you can glance from the screen to the keyboard just by moving your eyes instead of tilting your head up and down.

If you feel tension in your upper shoulders, stop working for a few seconds, take a deep breath and then let it all come out at once in a big sigh. As you exhale, completely release the tension in your shoulders and facial muscles. Let your body totally relax. It's like the old saying, "breathe a big sigh of relief." You put yourself in a state where you let go of tension and feel like a big load has just been lifted totally from your shoulders.

You can also drop your head down and place your hands over

your eyes and face and just relax in that position for a minute or so.

Take regular tension breaks. When you're concentrating deeply on something, set up some type of timer or alarm system that sounds a reminder every hour or half hour. You'll find short breaks actually increase your stamina, and they certainly help relax your shoulders and back.

I use a software program that sounds Westminster chimes every half hour as a reminder to get up, stretch, take a couple of deep breaths, walk around, and I come back to the word processor more refreshed. Otherwise, I would sit for hours at the keyboard and feel wiped out at the end of the day. People without a computer can buy a small digital clock or wristwatch that will sound every hour as a signal to take a short break. The break doesn't have to be long—a couple of minutes works wonders.

During the break you can rotate your head in circles, first one way and then the other. Then shake your shoulders and arms several times. After you've taken these regular tension breaks for a few weeks, it will become a welcome habit you'll be glad you picked up. Other muscle stress busters are given in Chapter 9.

The upper shoulder area is subject to buildups of fibrous gristle-like material after years of prolonged tension. A woman in Kansas had surgery to remove fibrous cartilage tissue which built up over the years from the habit of "hunching up" her shoulders during the day. This was in the days before massage became a legitimate means of easing muscle tension. Massage helps work out the knotted, locked muscles before scar tissue or lesions have a chance to form. Had she been able to get a mini-massage regularly, and learned some ways to relax her shoulders, she wouldn't have needed the surgery.

A condition called fibromyalgia, although it is not deforming or life-threatening, causes pain in the neck, shoulders, hips, knees, or back of more than 5 million Americans between the ages of twenty-one and fifty. Lack of energy, and depression are also symptoms of this disorder. More women than men suffer from fibromyalgia. Successful treatment includes massage, heat and exercise. Mild painkillers may be used. If pain persists in these areas, see a health professional for further treatment.

Bursitis is a common condition that results from too much pressure over a particular joint. It can strike any joint, such as elbow, knee or heel, although the arm/shoulder joint is the most common site of trouble. Bursitis is a painful irritation of the bursa, the little lubricating bag in the joint that's supposed to cut down friction between the tendons and bones. The condition may be brought on by injury to the joint or by repeated off-balance movements. Mini-massage can help reduce the pain of bursitis of the arm/shoulder joint by gentle stroking over the shoulder, upper arm and upper back.

Here are some other things you can do to relax your face, neck and shoulders. If you wear glasses, take them off. Let your lower jaw and shoulders drop to a relaxed position. If you notice your tongue up against your teeth or the roof of your mouth, bring it back to a normal resting position in the middle of your mouth. If you show tension in your forehead from wrinkling your brow, take the palm side of all four fingers and iron out the wrinkles, or "elephant skin" as one massage therapist calls them. Use both hands if you want.

Check the position of your head. Is it pitched forward so that you feel a tightness in the front of your neck and tension at the back of your head where the skull and neck meet? Is your head reared back so that you feel tension along the front of your neck from just under the chin to the collarbone? If you feel tension as a result of the position of your head or neck, don't force your head back or forward. Let it merely come up to a more centered resting position that feels comfortable to you. You may not think of doing this often at first, but after a while you'll find yourself remembering to check the position of your head several times a day.

You may have noticed that people who are feeling low or depressed tend to keep their heads bent down and watch the sidewalk as they move along. Bringing the head to an upright resting position helps break this negative habit. Once life starts "looking up," a person may begin to look up physically as well.

Frequently, the act of driving can cause shoulder tension. If you experience tension while driving, occasionally check the position of your head and arms and, especially, how tightly you are gripping the steering wheel. Are the muscles in your forearms tense and your knuckles turning white from the pressure of your grasp? If so, relax your hands and move them to a different position on the wheel. If possible, stop the car, get out and walk around it a couple of times. Check the tension in your face, head, neck and shoulders. Stretch, breathe deeply, rotate your head a couple of times and give your shoulders a few good shrugs. If you can't get out of the car, but are stopped at a traffic light, railroad crossing, stop sign or in a traffic jam, take both hands off the steering wheel and place them in your lap. Rotate your head once each way, shrug your shoulders a couple of times and take a deep breath and give a good loud sigh. Stretch your arms and shoulders, then drop them to a completely relaxed position. If you have a cassette or CD player in your vehicle, keep a favorite album with you and play it when driving or traffic begins to stress you out. Every little bit helps.

A hot shower is an excellent way to ease muscle tightness in your shoulders and upper back. You can direct the spray so that it targets these areas. If you have a pulsating shower head, the added force of the water is especially helpful. It's a good idea, if the area is really hurting, to alternate between hot and cool water, as the temperature change acts as a kind of pump to help remove the buildup of lactic acid in your muscles. Do about 30 seconds of cool water for every 3 minutes of hot. I like to end a shower with hot water for the relaxation it gives. Some people, however, like to end with cold water for the stimulation and energy it gives. Find out which order works best for you and do it that way. A soak in a hot bath, hot tub, Jacuzzi or sauna also helps to relax these muscles and reduce tension.

MASSAGE POSITION

A mini-massage on the upper back and shoulders can be done with the receiver in any of several positions. The person receiving a mini-massage on this area may leave his or her shirt or blouse on, although any necklaces or chains should be removed.

It is probably easiest and most effective to have the receiver sit in a chair, leaning forward, with his head resting on a pillow placed on an adjacent table. The shoulders and upper back are at a good angle for firm working pressure in this arrangement. Have the person either place his arms on the pillow or let them hang loosely by his sides as you work.

Giving a shoulder and upper back mini-massage on a massage table is fine, too. When using a massage table, it's probably better to have the person remove his or her shirt or blouse, as the front of the garment will be pinned by the body.

The massage chair gives great access to the neck, shoulders and back. (See illustration on page 54.) It's actually more comfortable than it looks. A complete illustration of the massage chair is shown under Massage Accessories in Chapter 8.

You can even give a mini-massage on the shoulders when the receiver is standing up, although this is the least effective position, and I don't recommend it. In the standing position, the receiver's body sways and moves when you apply pressure.

If you're giving the mini-massage on the floor, be sure the area is well padded for the comfort of both the giver and receiver. A thick carpet helps, but if the floor is bare, or thinly covered, you can spread a thick blanket, comforter, air mattress, foam rubber pad or even a sleeping bag on the floor. The receiver can place his arms alongside the body or folded underneath a pillow, with his head resting on the pillow—whatever is more comfortable. Many people find kneeling on the floor becomes uncomfortable very quickly. If the giver needs extra padding for his knees, he can use a regular pillow or cushion to kneel on.

If your knees, back or shoulders tire rapidly, there are ways to reduce your discomfort and still give a mini-massage with good results for the receiver. The main thing to remember is to keep your shoulders as relaxed as possible, whatever the receiver's position.

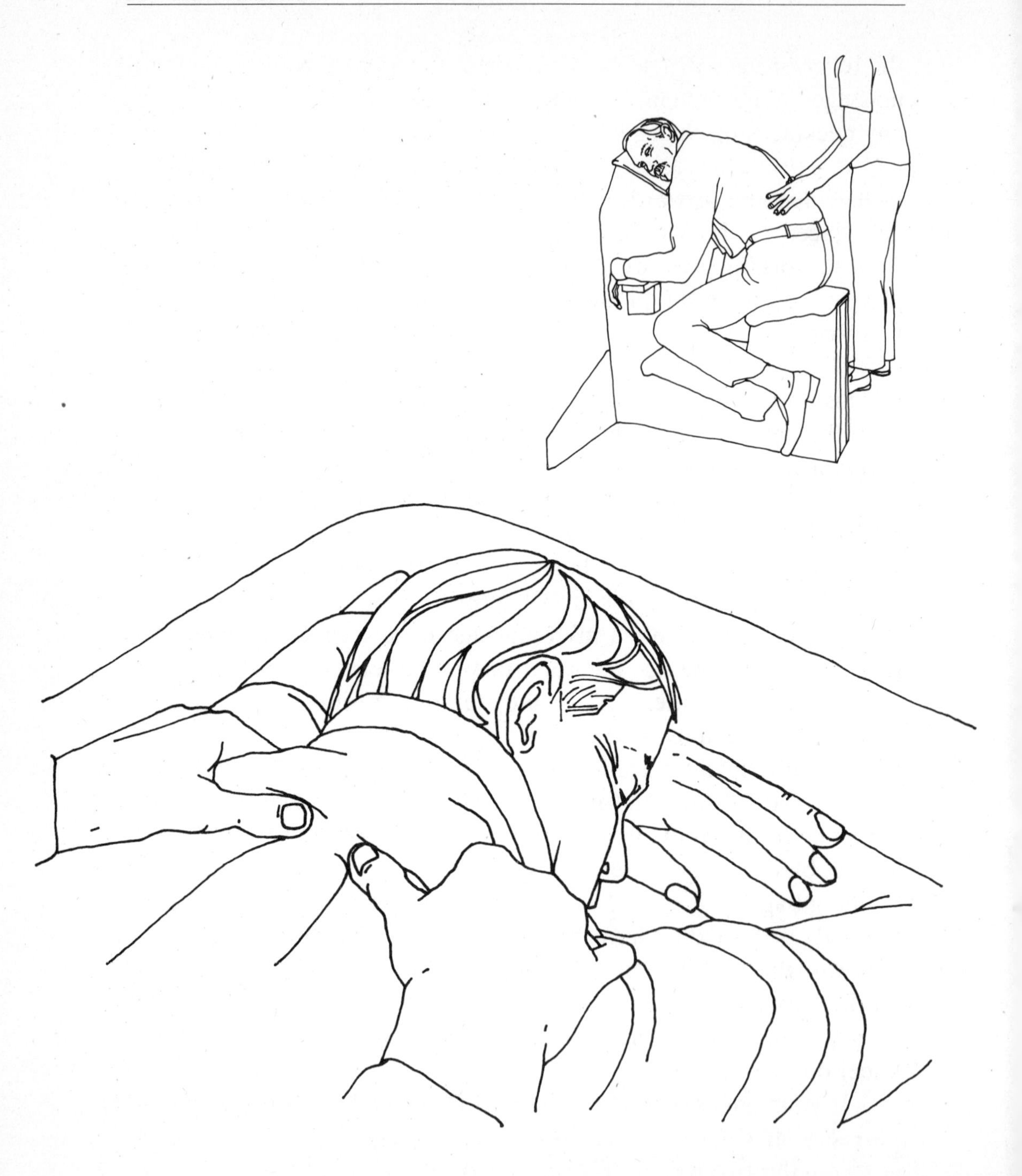

Your arms should not be stiff or your shoulders hunched up almost to your ear lobes. This is a sure way to wear yourself out—fast! It is better in this situation to sit alongside the receiver and reach over to do the movements, while still keeping your arms and shoulders relaxed. Also some of the tension you feel can be transmitted to the receiver.

At the end of a mini-massage you should always rotate your head and shake your shoulders and arms a few times to relax the upper part of your body. Do this even if you are going to change roles and receive a mini-massage yourself.

SHOULDER AND UPPER BACK MOVEMENTS

UPPER RIDGE OF SHOULDERS

Placed one hand over the top of each shoulder, with the thumbs on the back side and the fingertips on the front side.

Work back and forth from the end of the shoulder to the base of the neck with a gripping or clasping motion. As you move back and forth, vary the position of your thumbs to cover as much of the upper back as possible. Use firm pressure.

This movement is sometimes most effective when the receiver is sitting up straight in a chair as you can then give the shoulders a good working over.

If you're using one of the special massage chairs, try changing position so that your thumbs are on the chest side and your fingertips are on the back side.

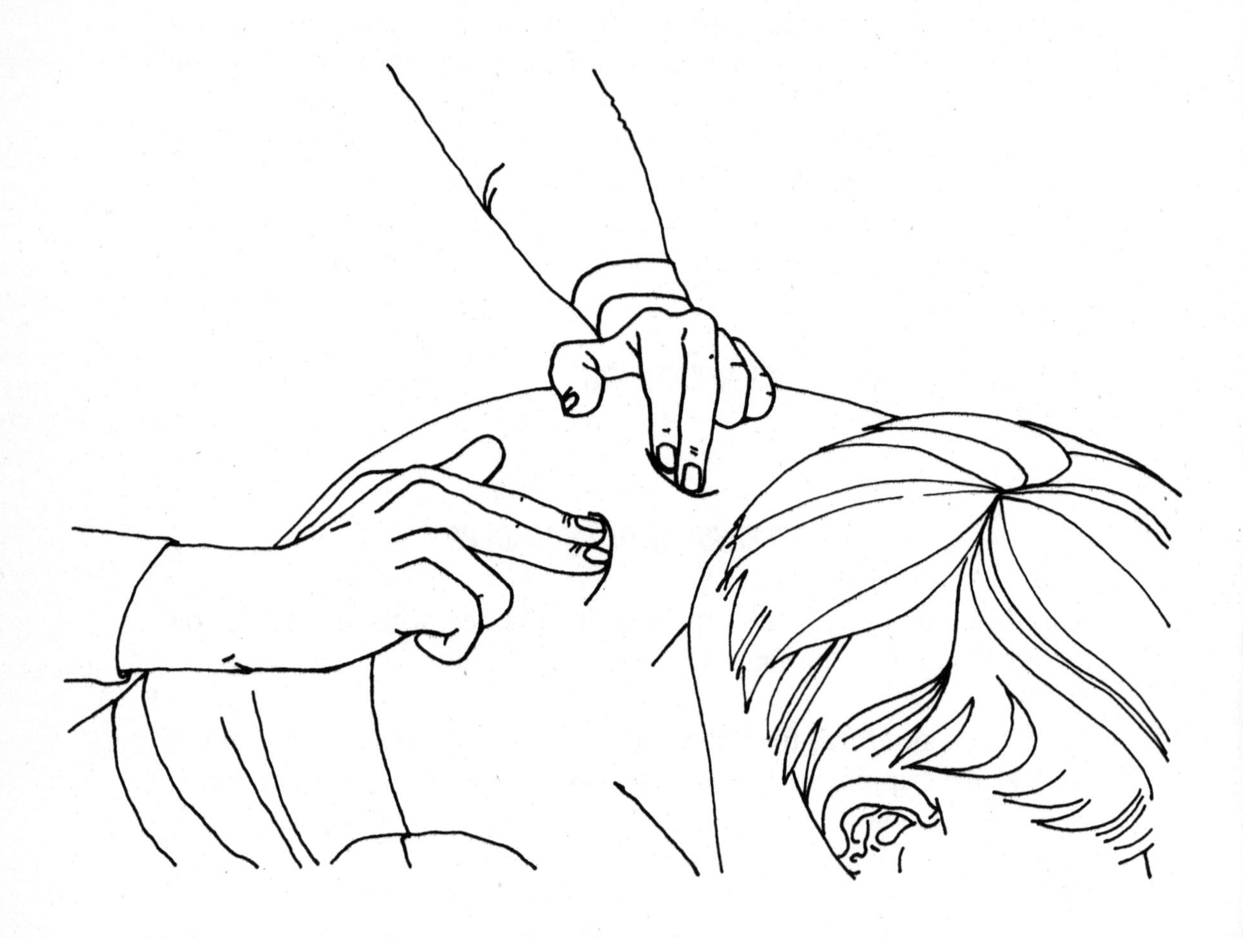

BETWEEN SHOULDER BLADES

Use two or three fingers of each hand to make circular or stroking movements in the area between spine and shoulder blades, from the bottom point of the shoulder blade to the base of neck. Use firm pressure.

Work all around this area as this region is a prime tension spot for many people.

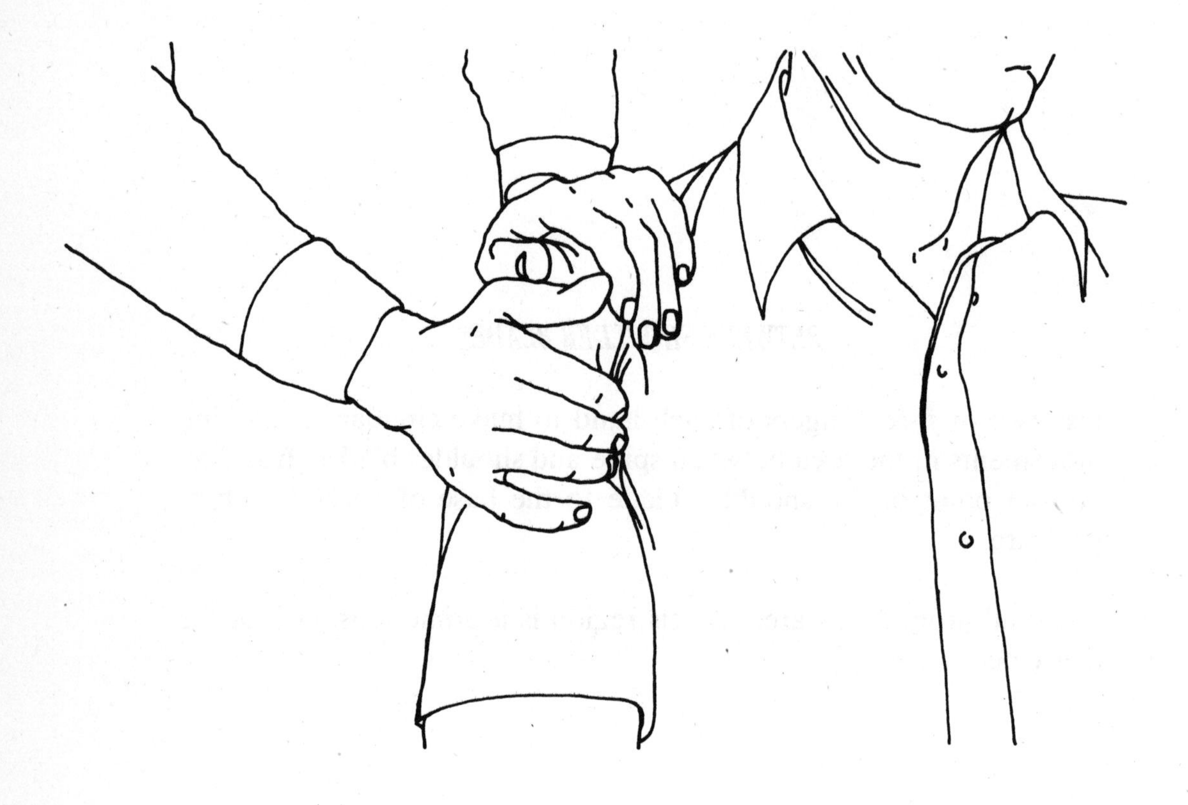

SHOULDERS AND UPPER ARMS

Place both hands over the round part of shoulder and upper arm. Use a firm gripping pressure to massage each shoulder. Work on one shoulder at a time.

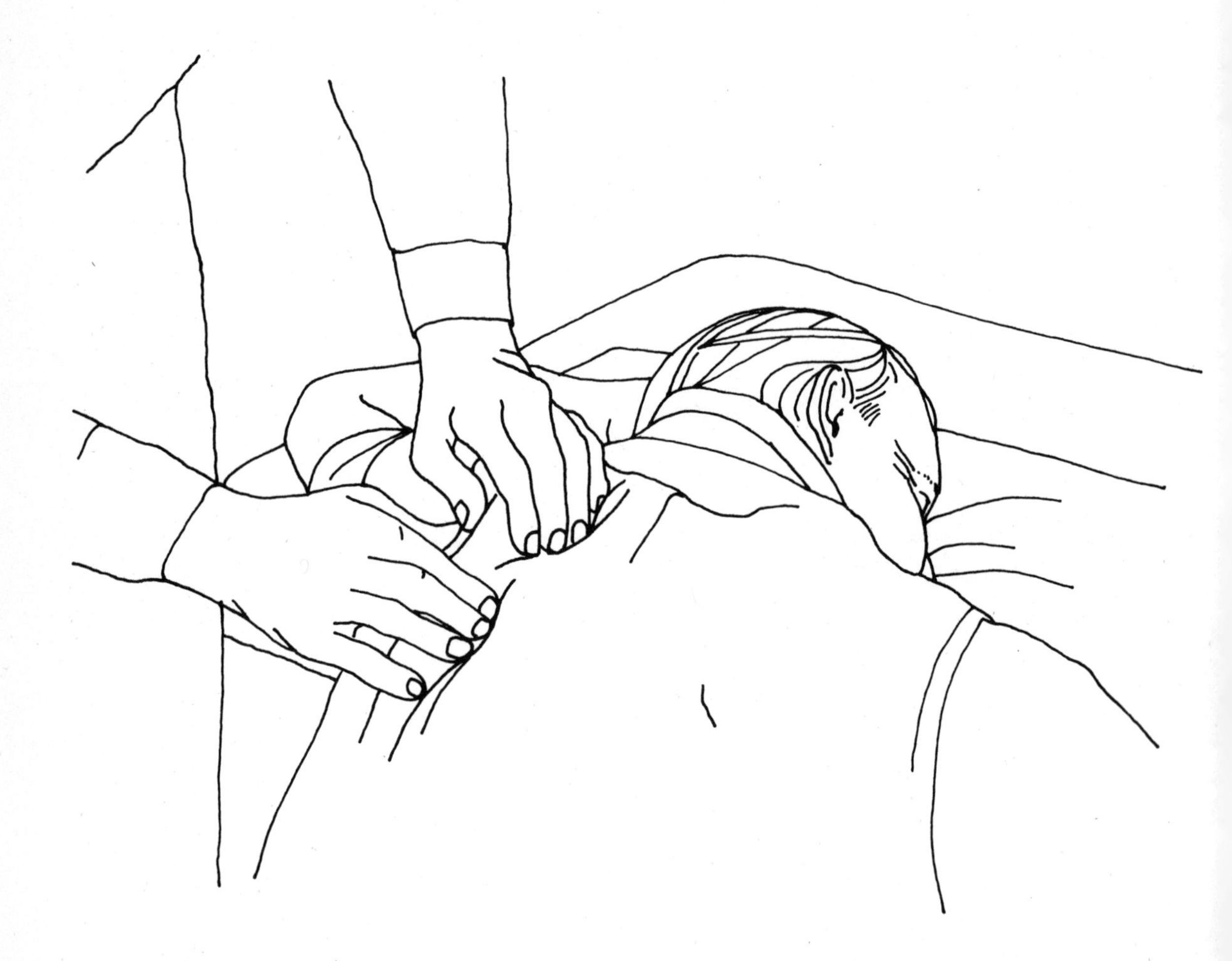

UNDER SHOULDER BLADES

Stand to one side of the receiver and place your fingertips just under the edge of one shoulder blade. Use medium pressure and dig in and under all along the inside edge of shoulder blade.

Change sides and work on the other shoulder blade.

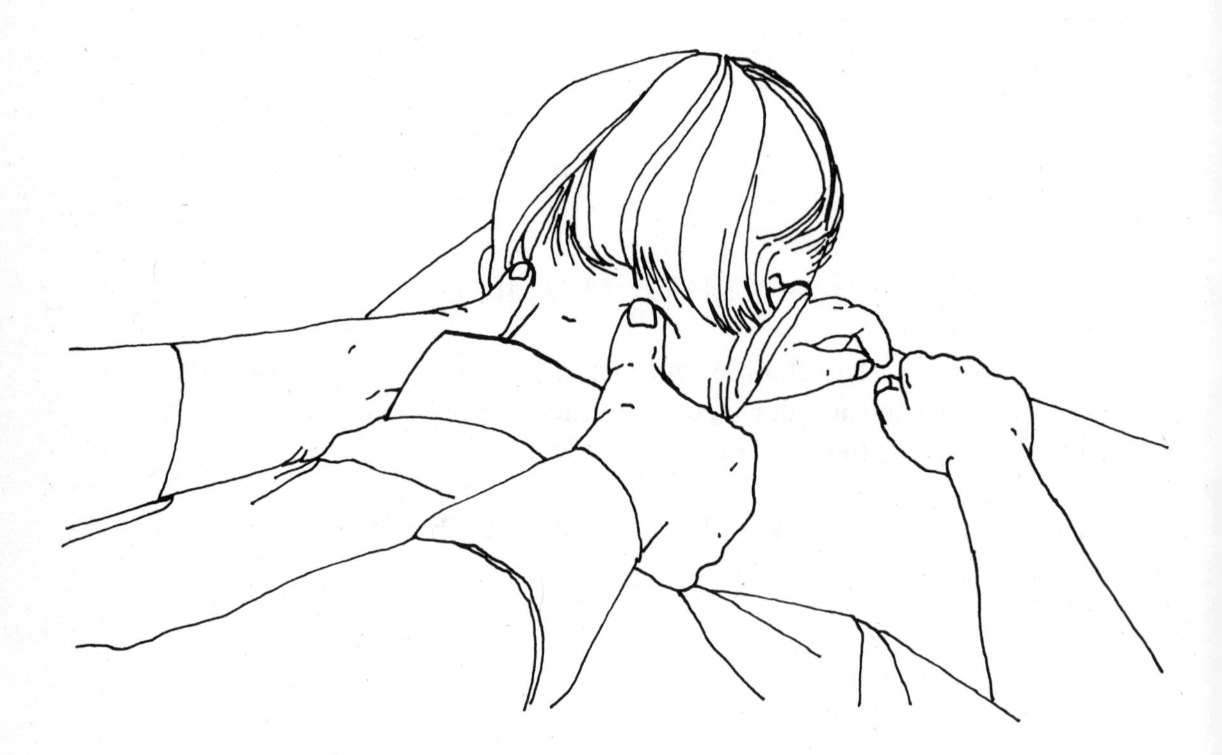

BASE OF SKULL

Place pads of thumbs in the notches just below the lower ridge of the skull. Let your fingers rest on the jawline for support but do not grip tightly. Apply steady pressure or pulsing movements with thumbs to this area. Use medium to firm pressure.

Work on this area for up to 3 minutes. This is where the large muscles of the upper back connect, via the neck, to the head. This movement is similar to Trepidation, page 47.

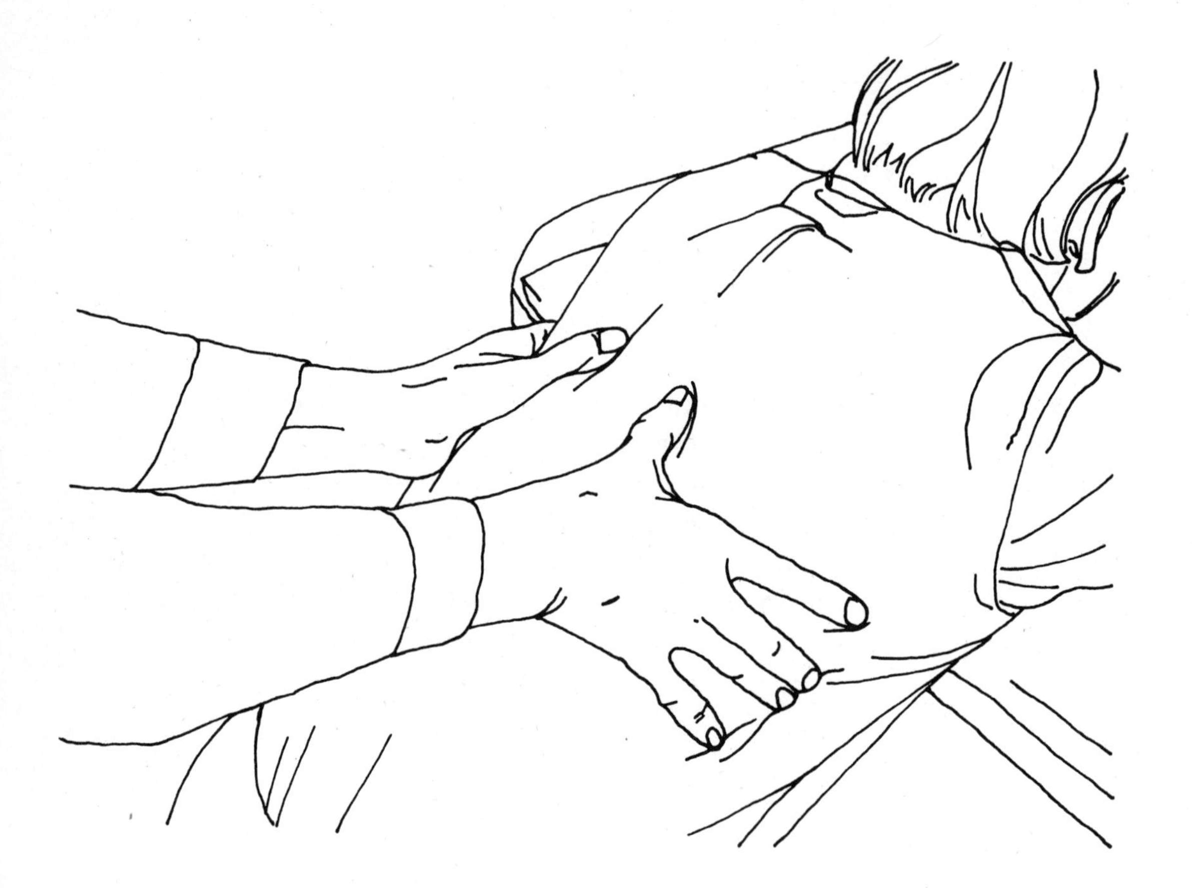

ACUPRESSURE

Use the ends of both thumbs to apply firm to heavy pressure on each side of the spine. Do not press directly on spine!

Work from the base of the neck down to the mid back and up again to the neck. Move thumbs about an inch at a time as you work up or down. Hold each position for a few seconds.

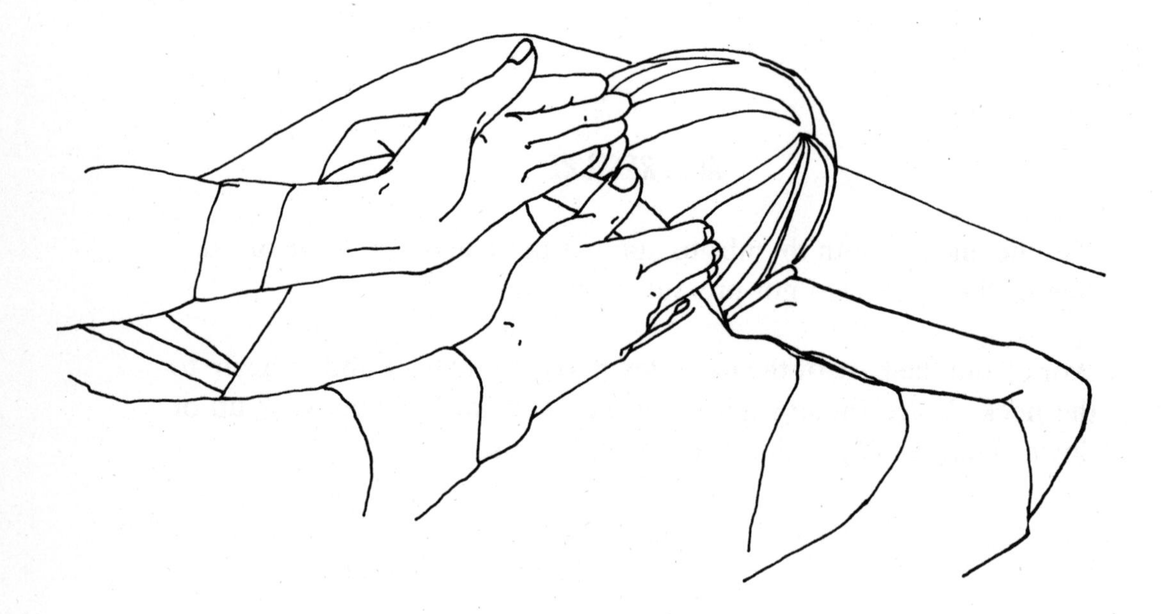

CHOPPING

Use the outside edges of the hands to make chopping movements across the shoulders and upper back. Keep fingers spread slightly apart. Do not hit spine.

Ask the receiver how much force he likes. Work back and forth several times.

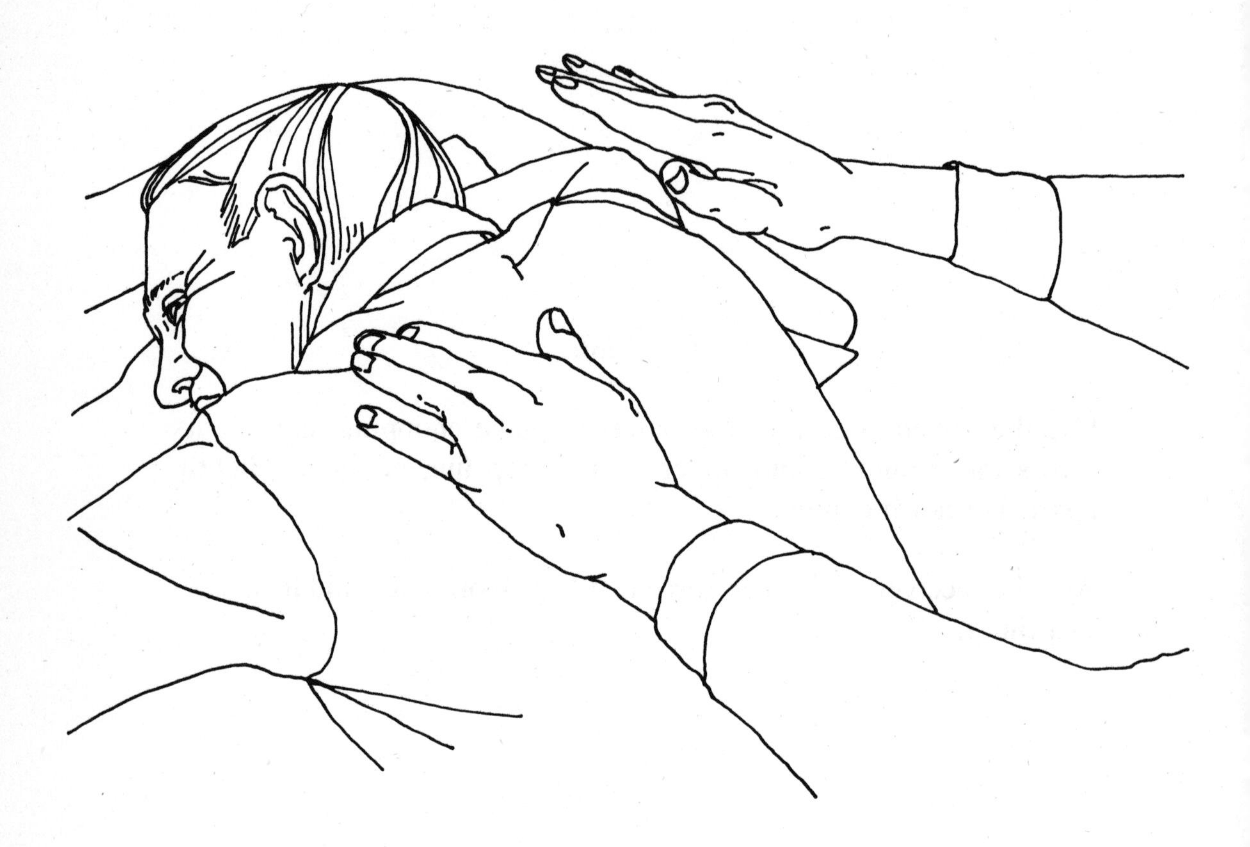

SLAPPING

Use the inside flat of each hand, palm and fingers, to deliver brisk, slapping movements over the whole upper back and shoulders. Do not slap directly on spine.

Vary the slap from light to heavy, depending on the preference of the receiver.

As a finishing touch, give a few light strokes all over the upper back and shoulders.

5

LOWER BACK

TENSION IN LOWER BACK

As I said at the beginning of this book, lower back pain affects one out of every two people at sometime during his or her life. It's part of the price we pay for being upright, walking human beings. Lower back pain results from a variety of causes: lifting heavy objects the wrong way, twisting too far, sleeping on too soft a mattress, using an improper chair, slumping down when sitting, standing on a hard floor all day, menstrual cramps, becoming emotionally upset, riding in a car for a prolonged time, or from many types of accidents. In *Mini-Massage* we're concerned with back pain that results mainly from muscle strain. Spinal injuries and slipped or ruptured discs present serious problems that need to be dealt with by a health-care professional. Although a mini-massage can help lessen some of the discomfort due to a spinal injury, it needs to be done lightly and only under the direction of a specialist.

For minor pains caused by muscle strain or tension, the use of a heating pad or heat lamp along with a mini-massage usually brings full relief. The hand-held heating lamp discussed in chapter 8, page 137, is good for the lower back as it radiates heat deep into muscle tissue.

LOWER BACK EXERCISE

Besides mini-massage and the use of heat, there is a quick, 2-minute exercise to help strengthen your lower back muscles and help prevent future lower back problems. First, lie down on the floor on your back. Grasp your legs just below the knees and pull them as close to your chest as comfortably possible. Hold for 5 seconds and release. Do this three times.

Next, while still lying on your back, place both legs flat on floor. Raise one leg and grasp it with both hands on the shin just below the knee. Pull your leg as close to your chest as you comfortably can. (This is similar to the first part of the exercise, except you do one leg at a time.) Hold for 5 seconds and release. Do this three times and then switch to the other leg.

Next, to balance out your back muscles it is necessary to strengthen your abdominal muscles. Remaining flat on your back, bend your legs at the knees and place both feet flat on the floor. Place both hands flat on your midsection and raise your upper body a few inches off the floor. Hold for 5 seconds and then return to the floor. Repeat 3 times. The next time you do the exercise, lie flat on your back with both legs flat on the floor. Place both hands on your midsection and raise your feet and legs a few inches off the floor. Hold for 5 seconds and then return them to the floor. Do this 3 times. You can feel your abdominal muscles tightening and getting stronger. Do these exercises several times a week.

Improper lifting of heavy objects is the major cause of lower back pain and injury. When lifting incorrectly, the load on your lower vertebrae can reach a tremendous 700 pounds per square inch. To lift a heavy object correctly, squat down in front of it, grab it underneath and then stand up slowly, keeping your back straight. Use your legs to push yourself up.

When you buy a new couch or chair, get used to sitting in it gradually by spending short times in it rather than an entire afternoon or evening. Similarly, break in a new car with short trips, if possible, to adjust to the new seat before you go on a long trip. Use pillows for back support if necessary in airline seats.

On long car trips stop every hour or whenever you come to a roadside park. Get out—stretch—and walk around the car a couple of times. When traveling with someone who can drive, switch places every couple of hours. If traveling by plane, train or bus, get up every once in a while and walk up and down the aisle. Avoid sitting for long periods of time and becoming tired or stiff.

When buying a new mattress and box spring, make sure they are the right firmness, although there's no surefire way to test a bed other than by sleeping on it. Many experts say that the firmer a mattress is, the better it is for your back.

Because of the change in the amount of support, any of these objects, when new, can throw your back out of whack and cause you some discomfort.

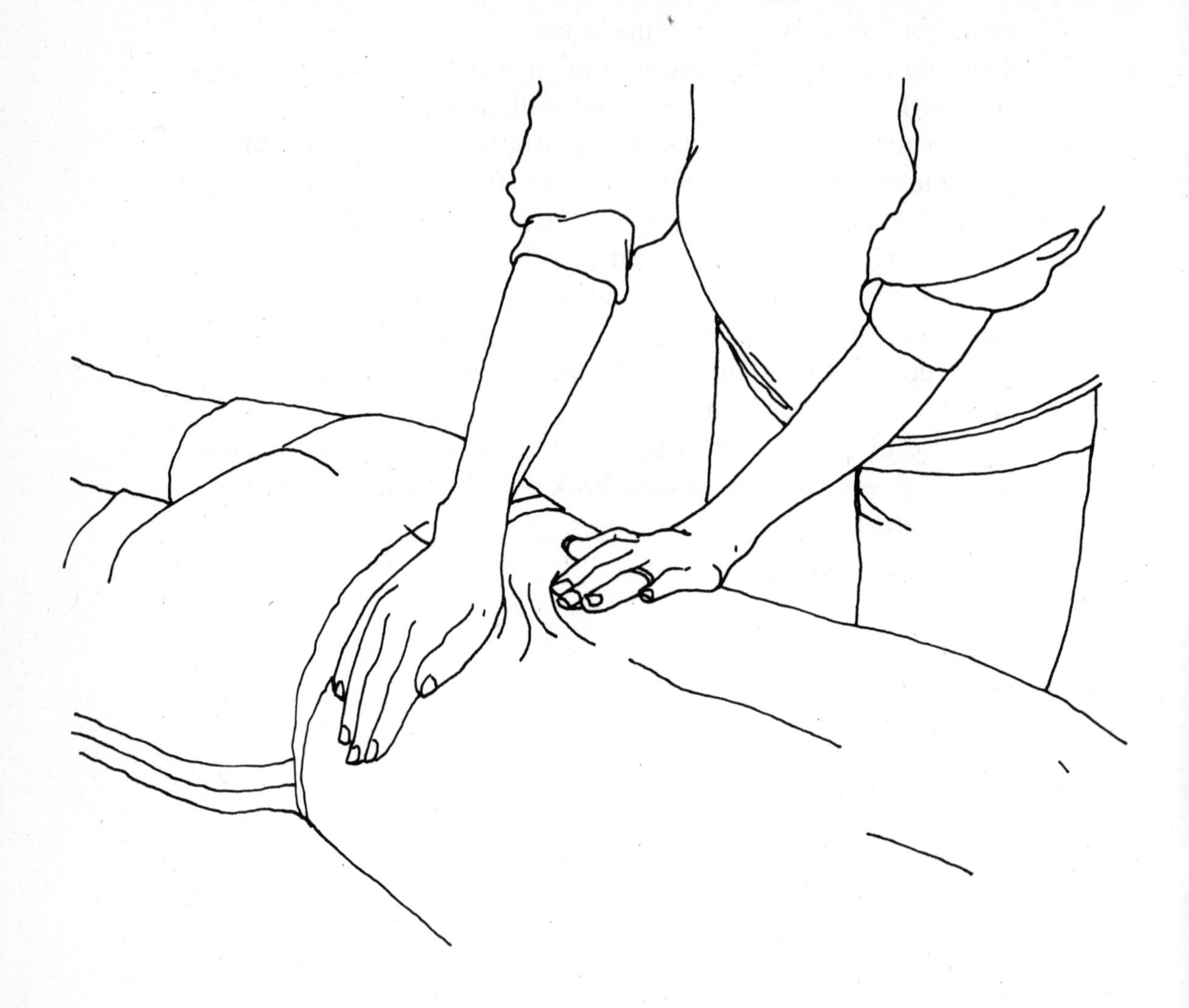

LOWER BACK MOVEMENTS

CRISSCROSS

Place one hand on the far side of the back and the other hand on the near side.

Applying firm pressure, pull toward you with the far hand and push away from you with the near hand. The skin on the back should wrinkle as you crisscross back and forth. Work from the mid back down to the pelvic bone and up again.

Do this movement several times.

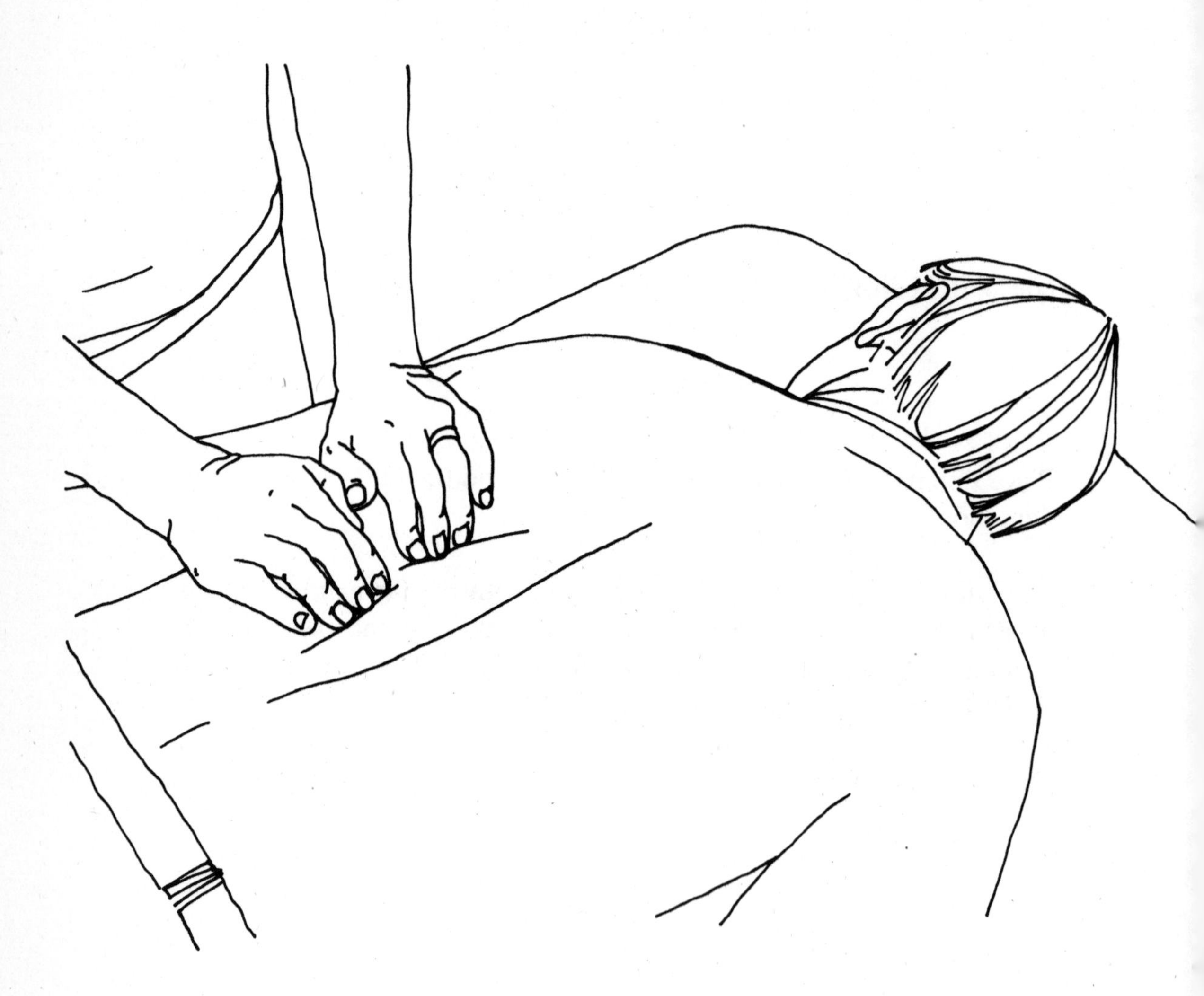

SPINE TINGLING

Place both hands on the side of the spine nearest to you. Place your fingers about ½ inch from the spine. Push down with firm pressure while at the same time pulling slightly toward you.

Work gradually from the upper back to the pelvic bone (ilium) and up again. Then change positions and do the other side.

As an extension of the spine tingling movement, knead the skin from the upper back to the pelvic bone by picking up folds of skin between the thumbs and first two fingers. Knead the whole area at least once.

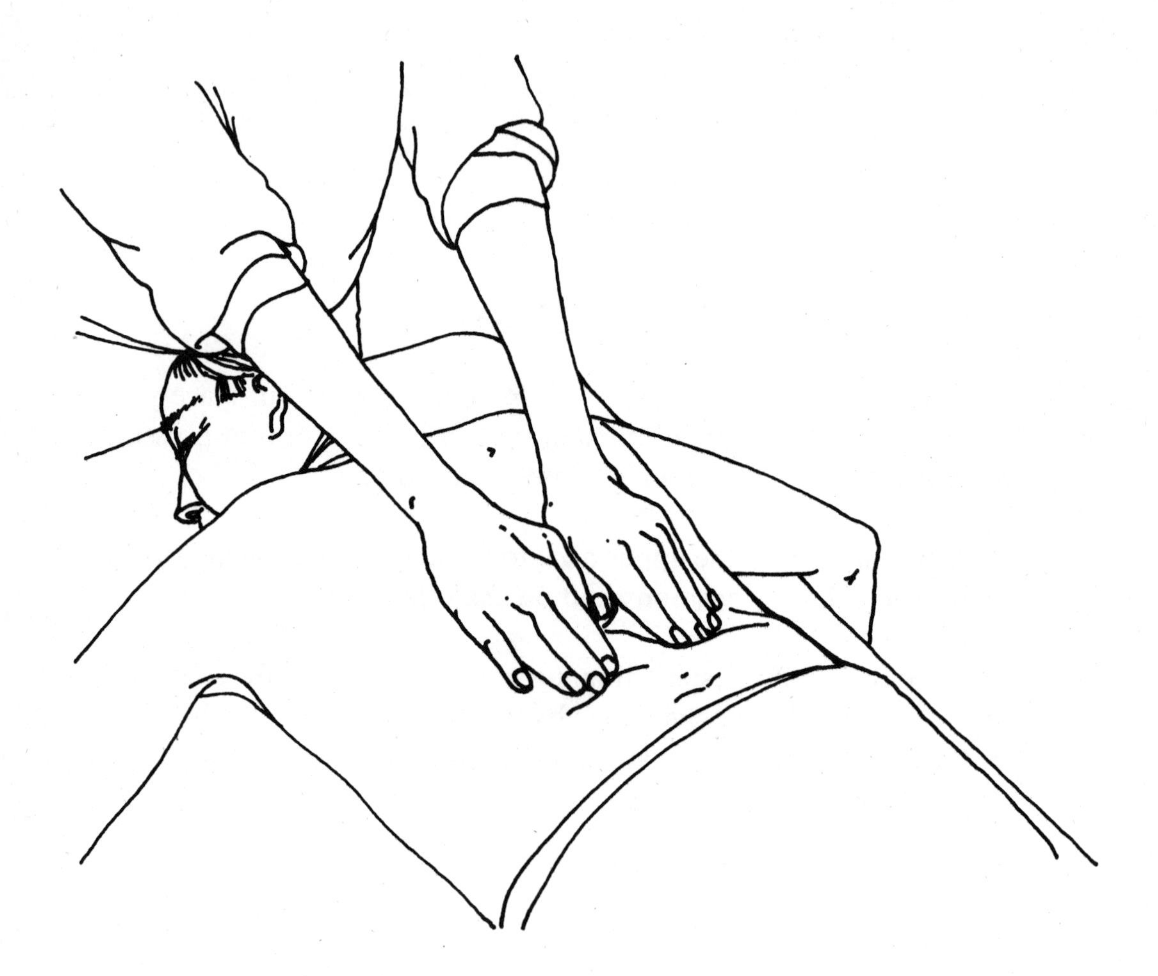

LONG STROKES

Position yourself at the top of the receiver's head. Place your hands flat between the shoulder blades and the spine, one on each side of the spine. Using the palms and heels of your hands glide down the back to the pelvic bone. Then slide your hands over so they run up along the rib cage and back to the starting position between the shoulder blades.

Use firm pressure and repeat several times.

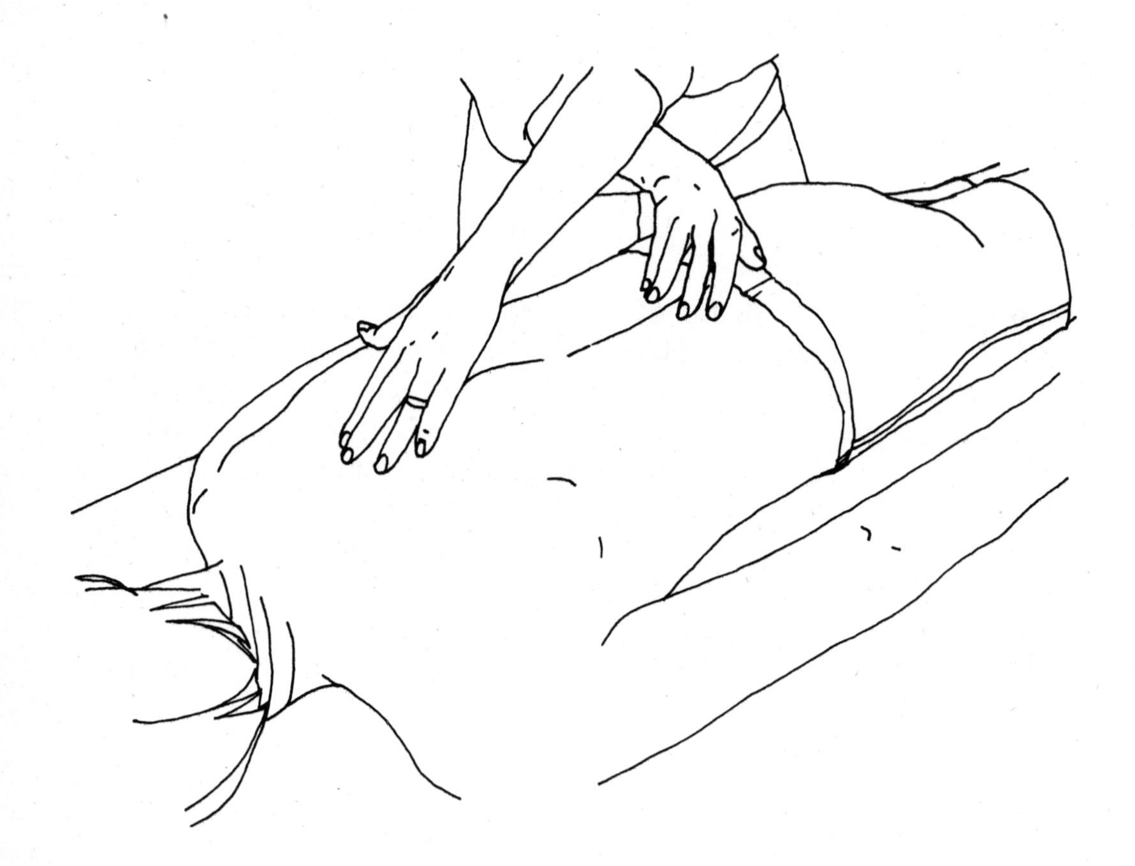

FAST BACKTRACKING

In this movement, you stimulate two of the most important paths of energy in the human body. Major acupressure and acupuncture points are located on each side of the spine. If there is excess tension in the back, these points will be painful when pressure is applied. The fast backtracking movement helps to release the energy blockages along the spine and rebalance the back muscles.

Spread the fingers of both hands slightly. Start between the shoulder blades with one hand and drag it along the spine down to the tailbone (sacrum). As one hand reaches the tailbone the other should be starting between the shoulder blades. Keep two fingers on each side of the spine.

Do this movement as rapidly as you can for up to 1 minute. This movement helps energize the nerve fibers in and around the spine. Use medium pressure.

As an added energizer, use the entire flat surface of the hands and fingers to briskly slap, working from the upper back down to the pelvic bone. This is the same as the Slapping movement, page 69.

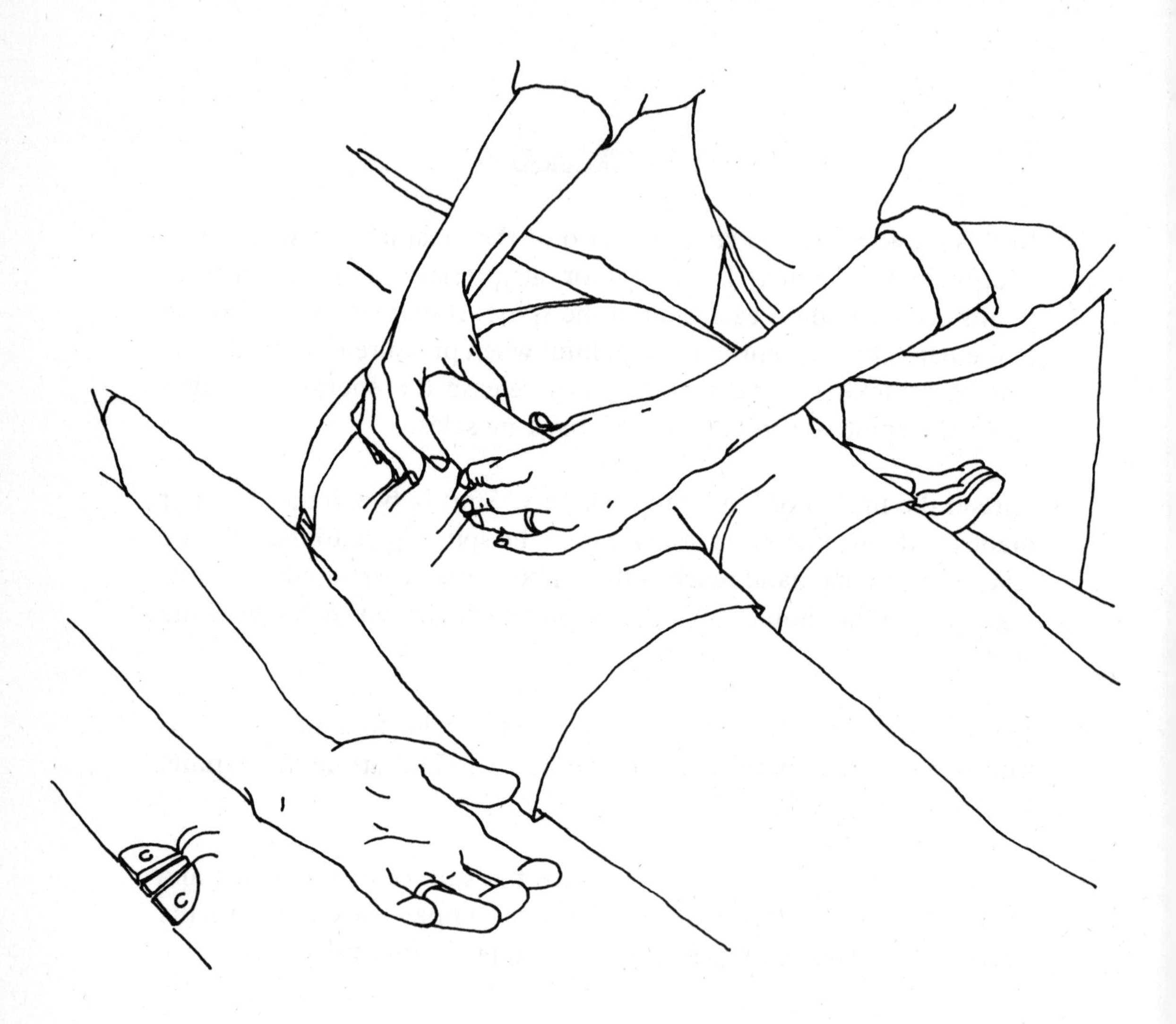

BUTTOCKS

Stand to the side of the body of the receiver and place both hands on one cheek of the buttocks. Grab as much skin as possible and use medium pressure to knead the tissue between your thumbs and fingers. Work over the entire buttocks.

Change sides, if necessary, to reach the other cheek.

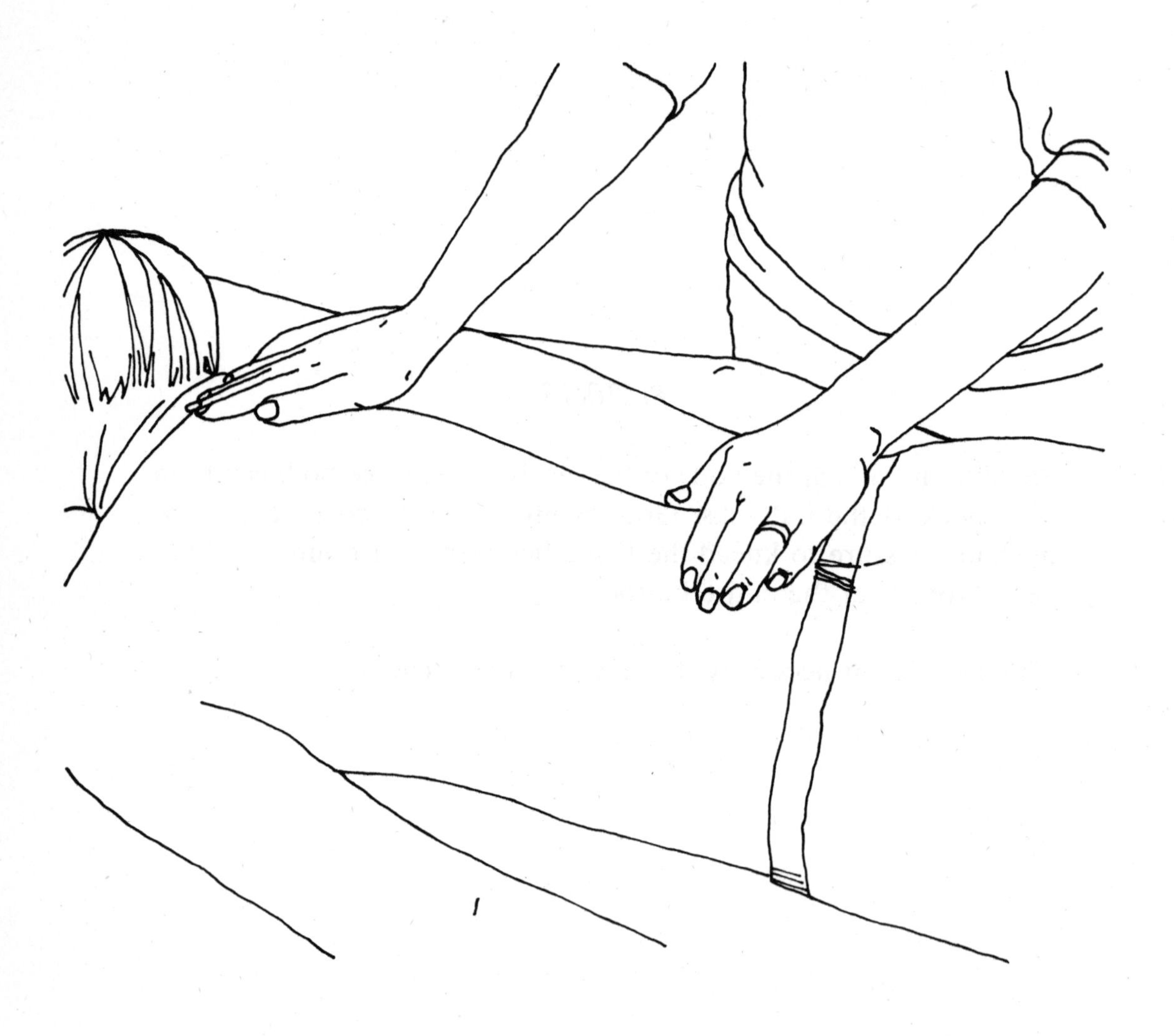

WARM HANDS/THERAPEUTIC TOUCH

Rub the palms of your hands together as rapidly as possible until they feel hot. Place one hand over the spine between the shoulder blades and one hand over the spine in the small of the back, just above the knobs on the pelvic bone.

Let the natural weight of your arms and hands rest against the receiver's body. Think of your hands as two powerful heat lamps transferring warm and soothing energy throughout the whole spinal area. Since this is the last movement, keep hands in place until it feels right to remove them. Then gently remove both hands at the same time.

6

STOMACH AND MIDSECTION

TENSION IN STOMACH AND MIDSECTION

The frontal region between the lower ribs and the pubic bone is a source of tension for some people. This area just below the navel is called the *hara* by Eastern teachers and is thought of as the focal point of life force energy. This mysterious energy is referred to as *ki* (kee), by the Japanese and *chi* (chee), by the Chinese. The *chi* or *ki* energy circulates through and animates your whole body. Those in the martial arts spend lots of time developing the skill to channel *ki* energy from the *hara* region to points in the hands and feet. Massage therapists using acupressure apply pressure to points along the *chi* meridians to relieve pain and promote healing.

We seldom talk about bowel and digestive problems, although they do exist. Many times you will find that people under stress automatically hold in and keep the *hara* region tight and tense. This tight, self-protective holding in of the midsection restricts the normal movement of the intestines and colon and can lead to constipation. It's as if the person is bracing her midsection to receive a blow from someone. (See Midsection, pages 121–123 of Chapter 8, for things to do to help relieve constipation.)

Emotional stress oftentimes manifests itself in the solar plexus region located just behind the pit of the stomach. People sometimes say things like, "I'm sick to my stomach of such and such," "I've got butterflies in my stomach," or "I feel like I'm tied up in knots" when referring to nervous problems in this region. The duodenum, which is the beginning portion of the small intestine where food exits the stomach, is a typical location for an ulcer. A tax accountant in New Jersey has his duodenal ulcer flare up during the first quarter of each year, when he's swamped with clients wanting their tax returns done yesterday.

A model in Paris gets a spastic colon every time she has to participate in a major showing of a new clothing line. A computer programmer in Santa Monica had to have a major operation to remove part of his colon because of a problem with nervous colitis. His office partner said the programmer was overly tense and that he didn't seem to know how to relax.

Many people suffer from acid indigestion. This may be an early warning signal of more serious problems later. Acid indigestion is a widespread problem, witness the number of advertisements and the number of products available for relieving excess stomach acid. It's not at all unusual to have an occasional digestive upset, which usually goes away after the stress has subsided, but constant pain connotes something more serious, and a health professional should be consulted. The time to deal with the problem is in the flare-up stage, before it becomes a chronic condition.

Several mini-massage movements serve to relieve tension in the midsection. Since you are working on a part of the body that's easy to reach, you can do this mini-massage on a massage table, sofa, bed or even the floor. There's no need for the person to take off all his or her clothing as the movements can be done through tights or by opening or pulling up the shirt, sweater or blouse and exposing the area from the ribs to the pubic bone.

Caution: Do not massage the intestinal area if pain is present. This might be a sign of appendicitis or some other serious problem and you should consult your doctor.

STOMACH AND MIDSECTION MOVEMENTS

COLON
(small circles)

Place one hand on the receiver's thigh or shoulder and the other on the area of the colon (large intestine) just above the right hip. Use the pads of the first three fingers and, applying medium-to-firm pressure, move slowly in small circles along the path of the colon—up the right side to the rib cage, follow just under the rib cage and down the left side toward the center of the pubic bone.

Always work from the right side to the left side as this is the path of digested food as it moves through the colon. Repeat several times, especially if constipation is present.

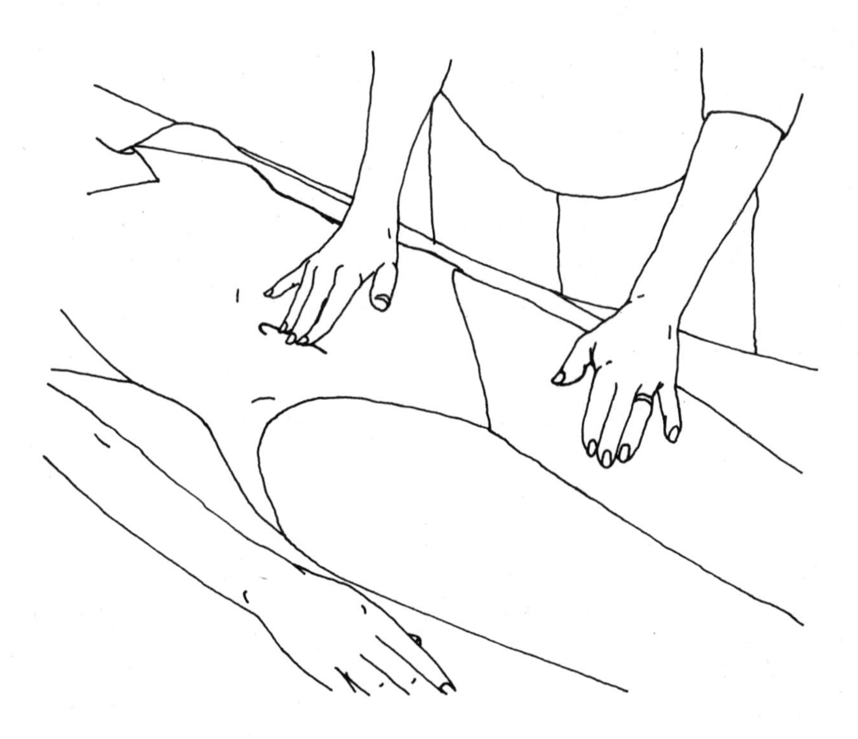

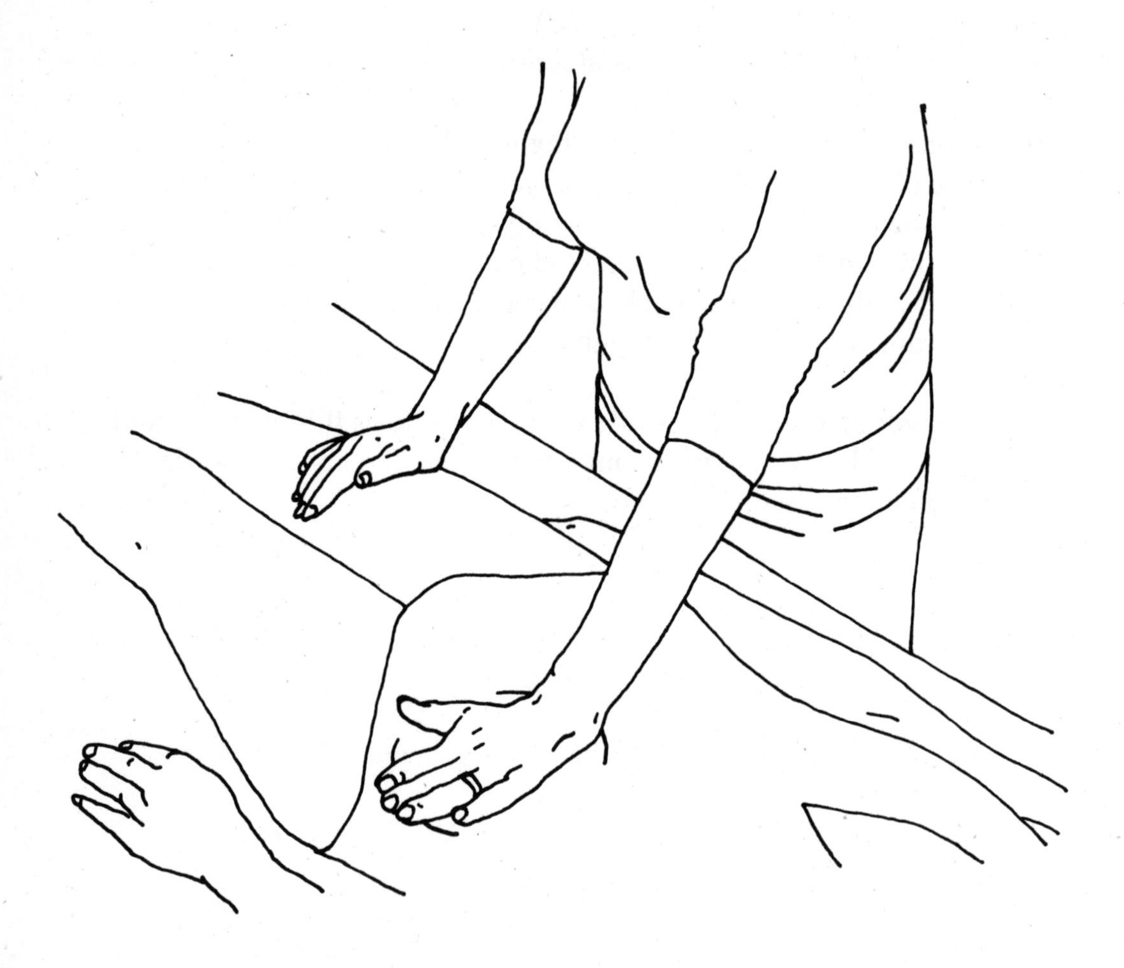

COLON
(large circles)

Place one hand on the receiver's leg or shoulder and the other on the right side of the intestinal area. Use the whole hand to slowly trace large circles around the colon and intestinal area, working always from the right side of the receiver's body to the left side. Use firm pressure and repeat several times.

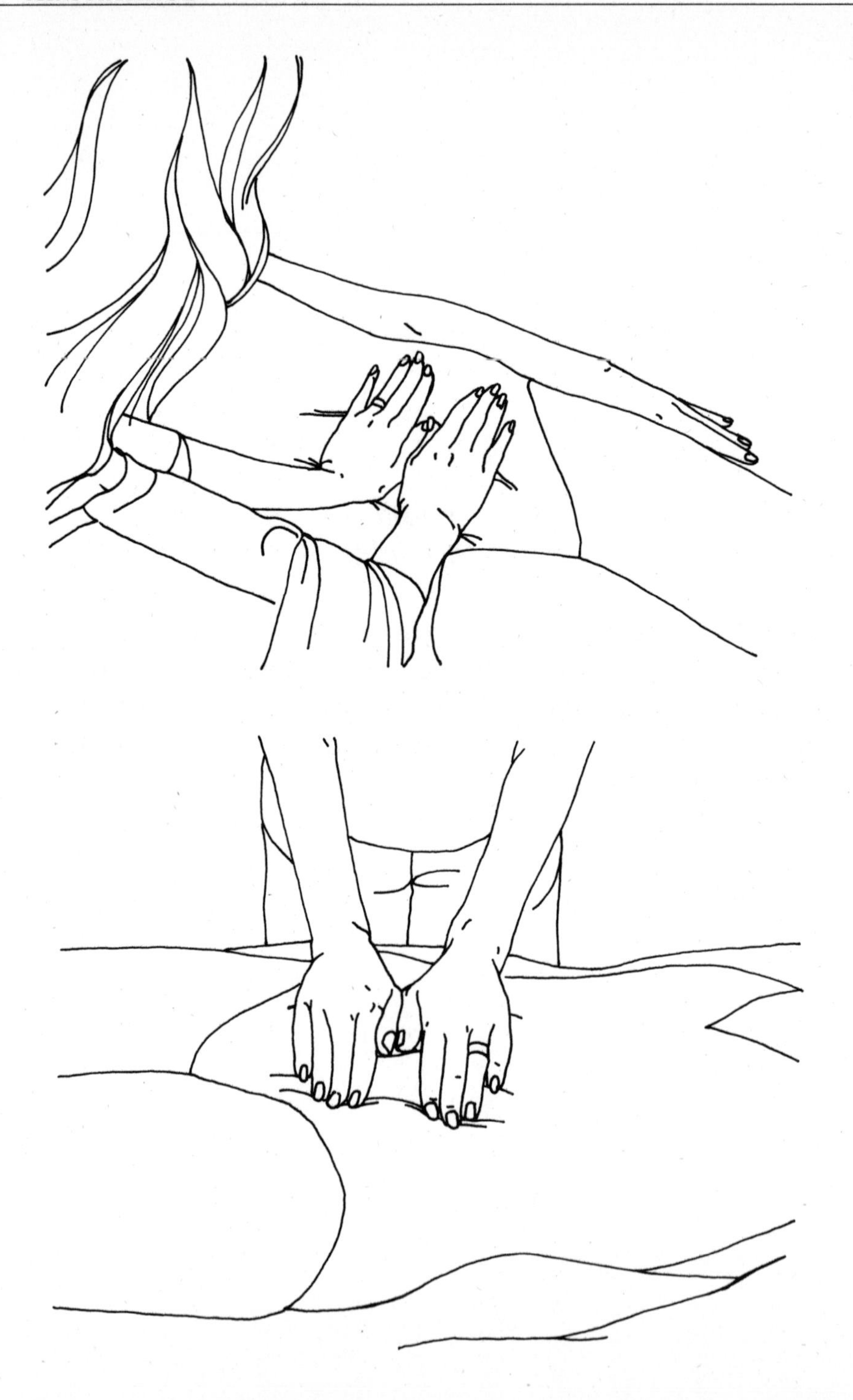

ROCKING HANDS
(pushing/pulling)

This is a two-part movement. For both parts, place your hands flat on the midsection between the lower edge of the rib cage and the upper edge of the pubic bone. The heels of your hands should be on the right side of the receiver's intestinal area, with your fingertips reaching toward the left side.

In the first part, use the heels of your hands to push the intestinal area away from you, using medium to firm pressure.

In the second part, use the finger pads of both hands to pull the intestinal area toward you. This is a rocking movement: push-pull, push-pull, push-pull as you go across the body.

Starting from the right side, push, then pull from the left side. Move hands slightly up or down each time so that you cover the entire midsection before going on to the next movement. Ask the receiver to elevate her knees with her feet flat on the table if deeper action is desired.

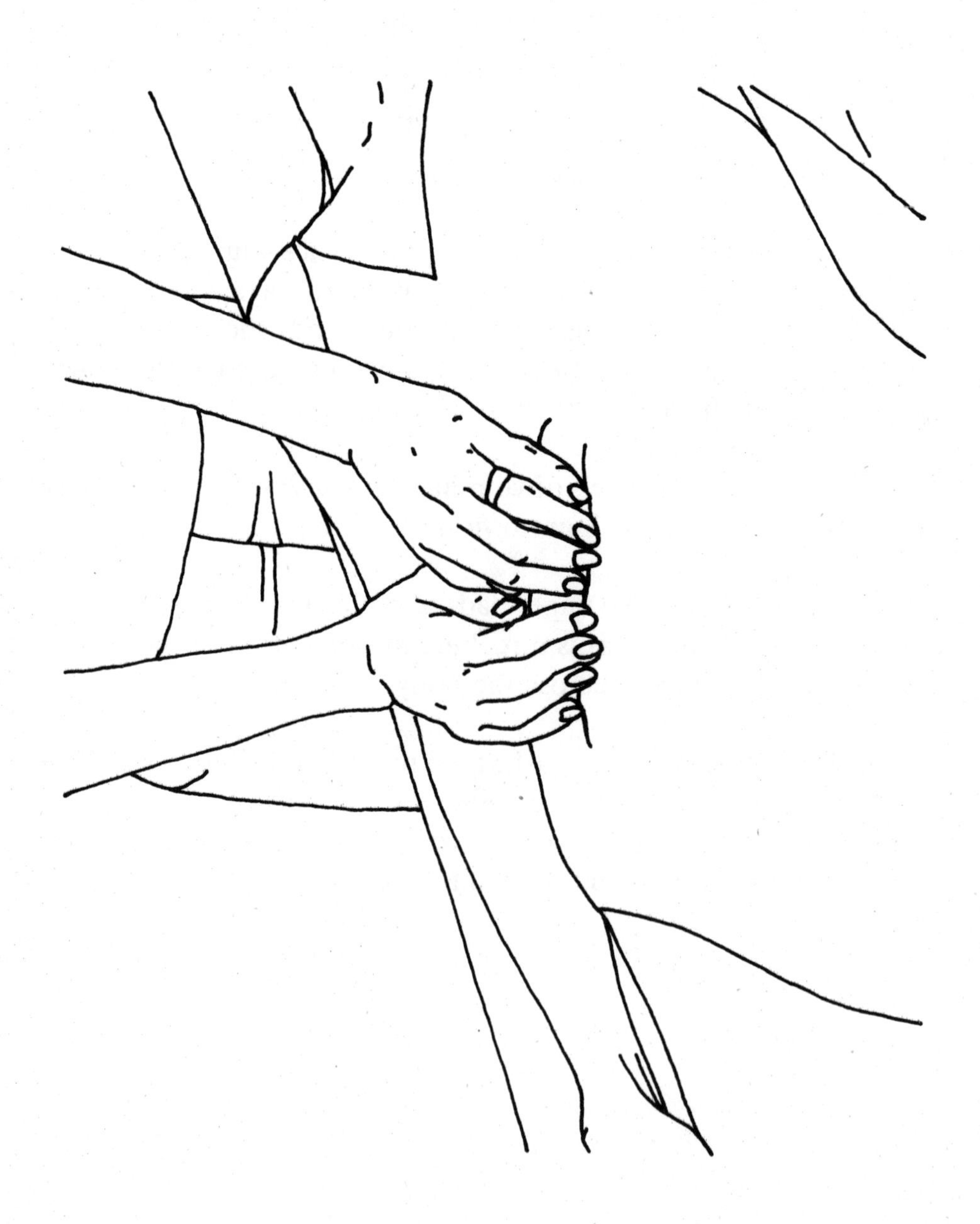

DIAPHRAGM/LIVER/GALLBLADDER

Position yourself on the right side of the receiver. Place the pads of your fingers just below the right rib cage. Creep along, slightly digging in and under the lower ribs, from the bottom of the rib cage to the upside-down V at the bottom of the breastbone. Work back again.

Change sides and work along the left rib cage. Use medium pressure and repeat several times.

Note: Do most of the work on the right side as that's where the liver and gallbladder are located. Do some of the work on the left side to keep the movement balanced.

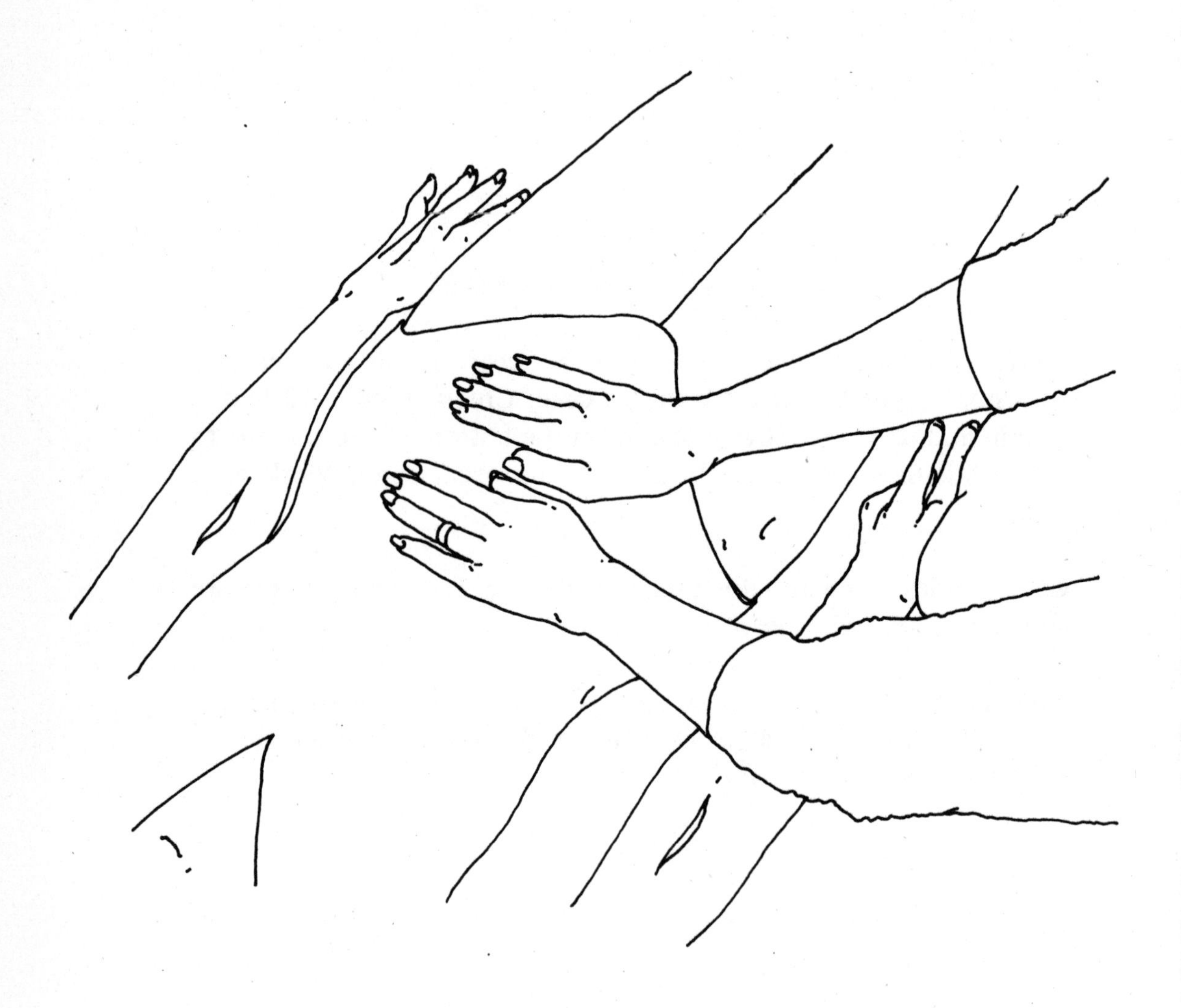

WARM HANDS/HEALING TOUCH
(horizontal)

Rub your palms together as briskly as possible until they feel hot. Place one hand just above the navel and one hand just below the navel. Keep the hands in a horizontal position.

Let the natural weight of your arms and hands rest against the receiver's body. Think of your hands as two powerful electric generators sending calming and healing energy throughout the whole digestive area. Keep hands in place for at least 1 minute and gently remove both hands at the same time when it feels right to do so.

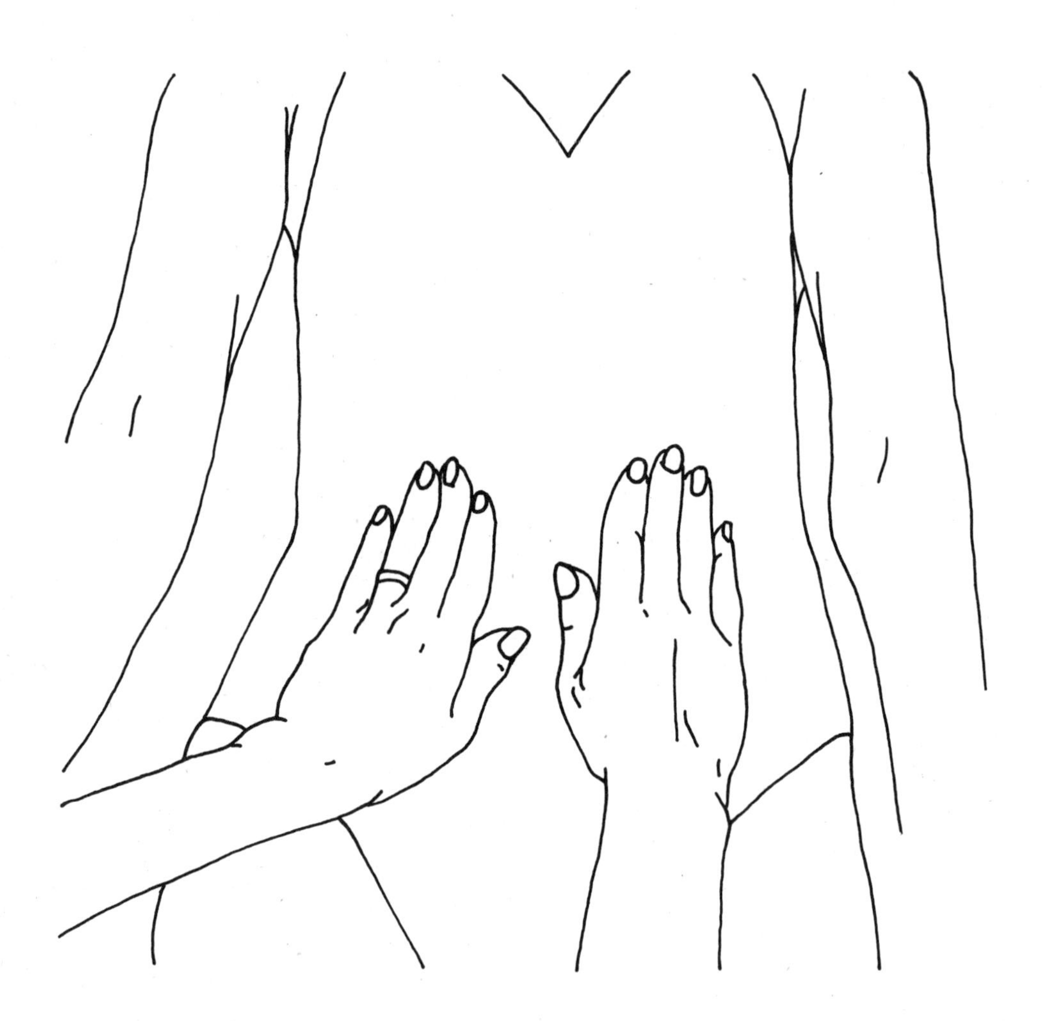

WARM HANDS/HEALING TOUCH
(vertical)

Again, rub the palms of your hands together until they feel hot. Gently, place a hand vertically on each side of the navel.

Let the natural weight of your arms and hands rest against the receiver's body. Think of your hands as two powerful heat lamps transferring warm and soothing energy throughout the whole digestive area. Since this is the last movement, keep hands in place for at least 1 minute and gently remove both hands at the same time when it feels right to do so.

7

LEGS AND FEET

TENSION IN LEGS AND FEET

Feet, knees and legs take a pounding in the modern world. Cities spawn thousands of miles of concrete sidewalks, and in most office buildings, department stores, shopping malls, service stations, airport terminals and restaurants, we walk on bare concrete floors or ones with tile or a thin layer of carpet covering the concrete.

A foot mini-massage resembles the ancient practice of foot reflexology, which has gained popularity in recent years. The Chinese originally defined and located energy and sensation pathways called nerve meridians. Reflexologists believe that all the nerve meridians for the whole body tie into parts of the feet from the ankle to the toes. Some people use reflexology on themselves as a way to start their day. This balances out the meridians and helps locate potential trouble spots. Although no hard scientific evidence exists for the theory behind foot reflexology, many people say it helps reduce overall body tension. If you're interested, there are several books available including Mildred Carter's classic, *Helping Yourself with Foot Reflexology*, and a more recent book by Nicola M. Hall, *Reflexology*.

An airline ticket agent in Toronto tried several different kinds of massage, from hour-and-a-half full-body massages to mini-massages on various parts of his body, to help relax after a day of being on his feet. He finally settled on a 20-minute foot massage as working best for him, since he couldn't get comfortable with a total massage, and mini-massages on areas other than his feet just didn't relax him enough. He said a good foot massage lowered muscle tension throughout his whole body.

FOOT HEALTH

You can now buy a specially designed shoe for almost every type of sport or activity. There are different types for runners, joggers, walkers and hikers, mountain climbers, bicyclists and bowlers. Special sports models for baseball, football, basketball and tennis are available for everyone. The proper shoe for the activity you're engaged in can make a big difference in your foot and leg comfort.

The knees are a big target injury site for joggers and runners. The owner of a health food store on Maui, Hawaii, spent every evening jogging a minimum of 10 miles with his wife, even though he was in constant pain. When asked how he planned to deal with the pain he was having, he replied, "Oh, I'm scheduled for knee surgery next week." When asked how long it had been since he jogged last, he said, "Yesterday. I wouldn't think of stopping my jogging routine." Well, he had to stop his jogging routine while he recovered from the surgery. Obviously, this man is an extreme case. Had he listened to what his knees were telling him as he jolted them, running on the hot asphalt roadways on the side of Mount Haleakala for better than two years, he probably wouldn't have needed the surgery.

Although it's especially true for the legs, knees and feet, by listening to the pain in all your muscles, joints and tendons you can often tell when something you're doing is causing too much stress on some part of your body. You can help prevent further problems merely by laying off that activity for a few days and then resuming the activity on a more moderate scale. It's hard for a muscle, joint or tendon to heal if it is being overworked or abused every day.

LEG AND FOOT MOVEMENTS

CROSS CALF

Have the receiver lie on his stomach. Place both your hands on calf area of his leg. Use your thumbs to iron the calf muscle in an upward, outward movement from the center of the leg to the outside. Work across the muscle, all up and down the calf. Use medium to firm pressure, and work each calf several times.

This can also be done on the upper part of leg.

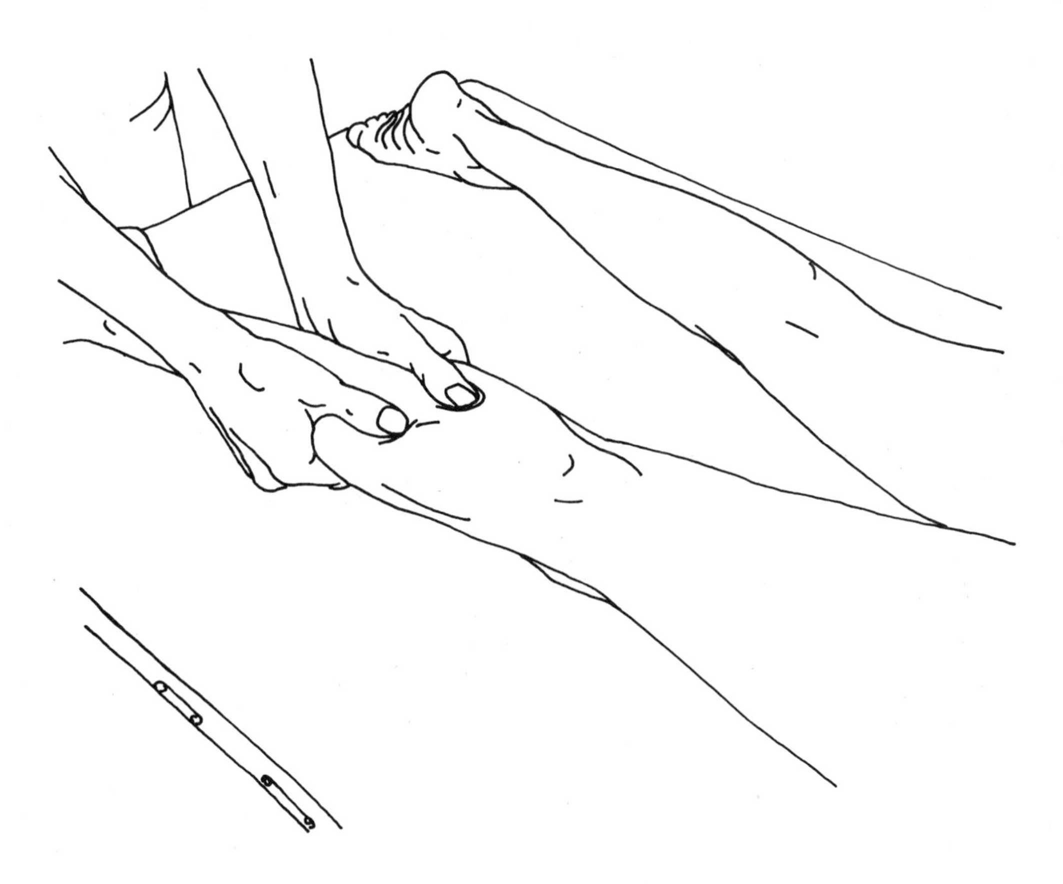

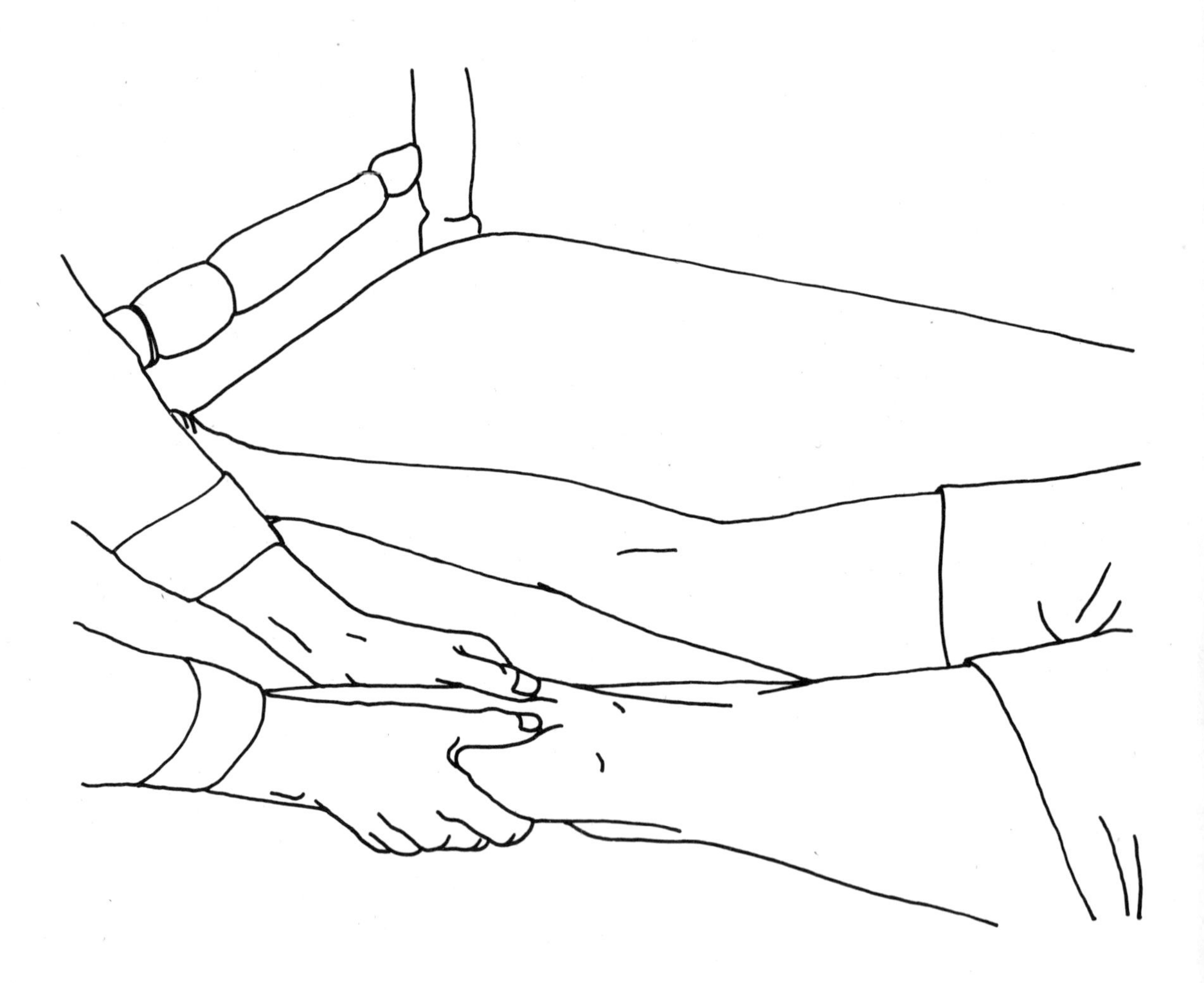

LONG STROKES
(back of legs)

Apply a small amount of oil or massage cream to your hands. Starting at the top of the receiver's leg, place both hands on one leg and draw them down to the ankle.

Maintain a firm pressure during each stroke. Make several strokes, covering the back of each leg.

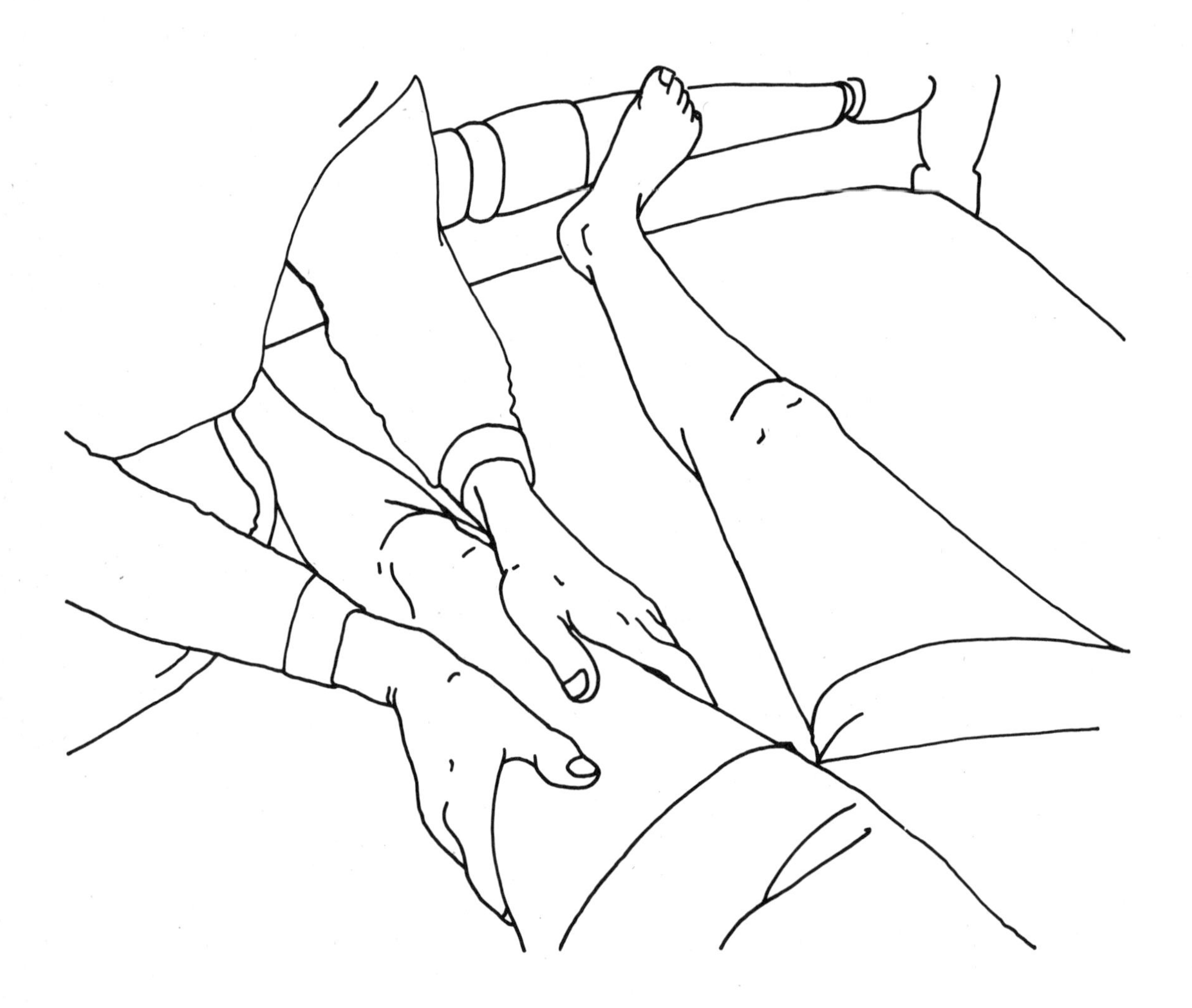

LONG STROKES
(front of legs)

Have the receiver roll over onto his back. Apply a small amount of oil or massage cream to your hands. Starting at the upper thigh, drag hands down one leg to the foot. Maintain a firm pressure during each stroke. Make several strokes, covering the front of each leg.

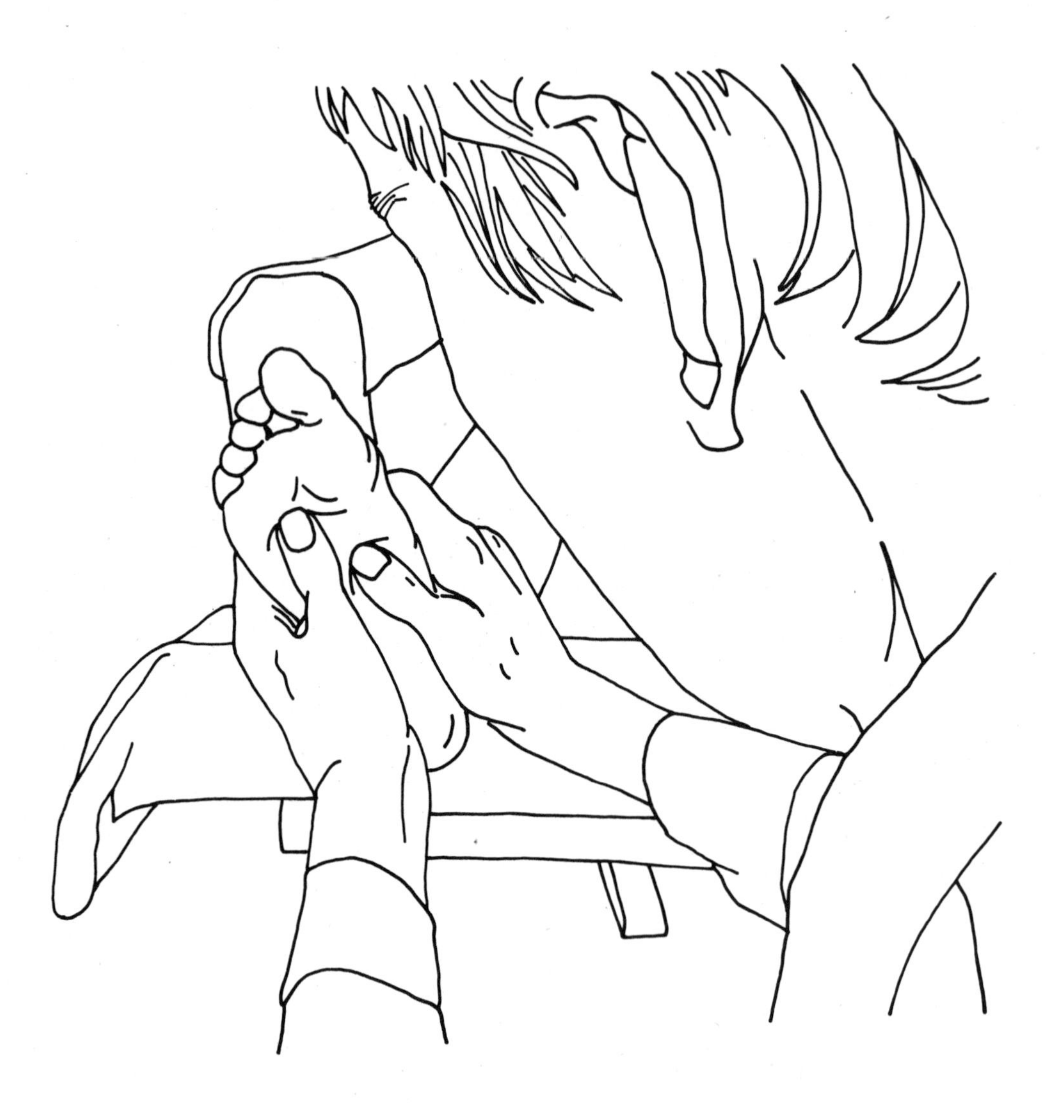

THUMBS ON SOLES

Place both thumb pads on one foot with your fingers around and on top of the foot. Use a firm to heavy pressure. Work from the base of the toes to the bottom of heel several times. Use a kneading or pulsing motion. Dig into the tissue to stimulate the entire sole of the foot.

Work each foot from top to bottom and back.

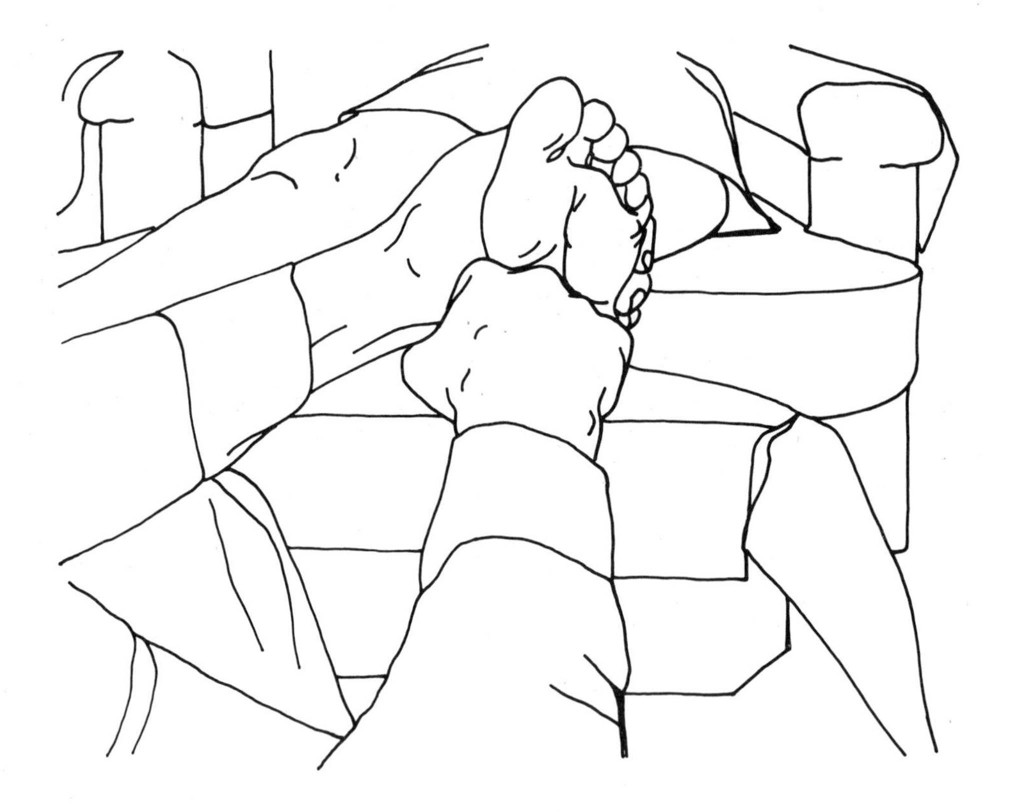

KNUCKLES ON SOLES

Make a tight fist and, with a twisting motion, work knuckles into the sole of the foot from the toes to the heel. Work each foot from top to bottom and back several times. Brace the foot with your other hand so that the receiver does not have to push against your pressure.

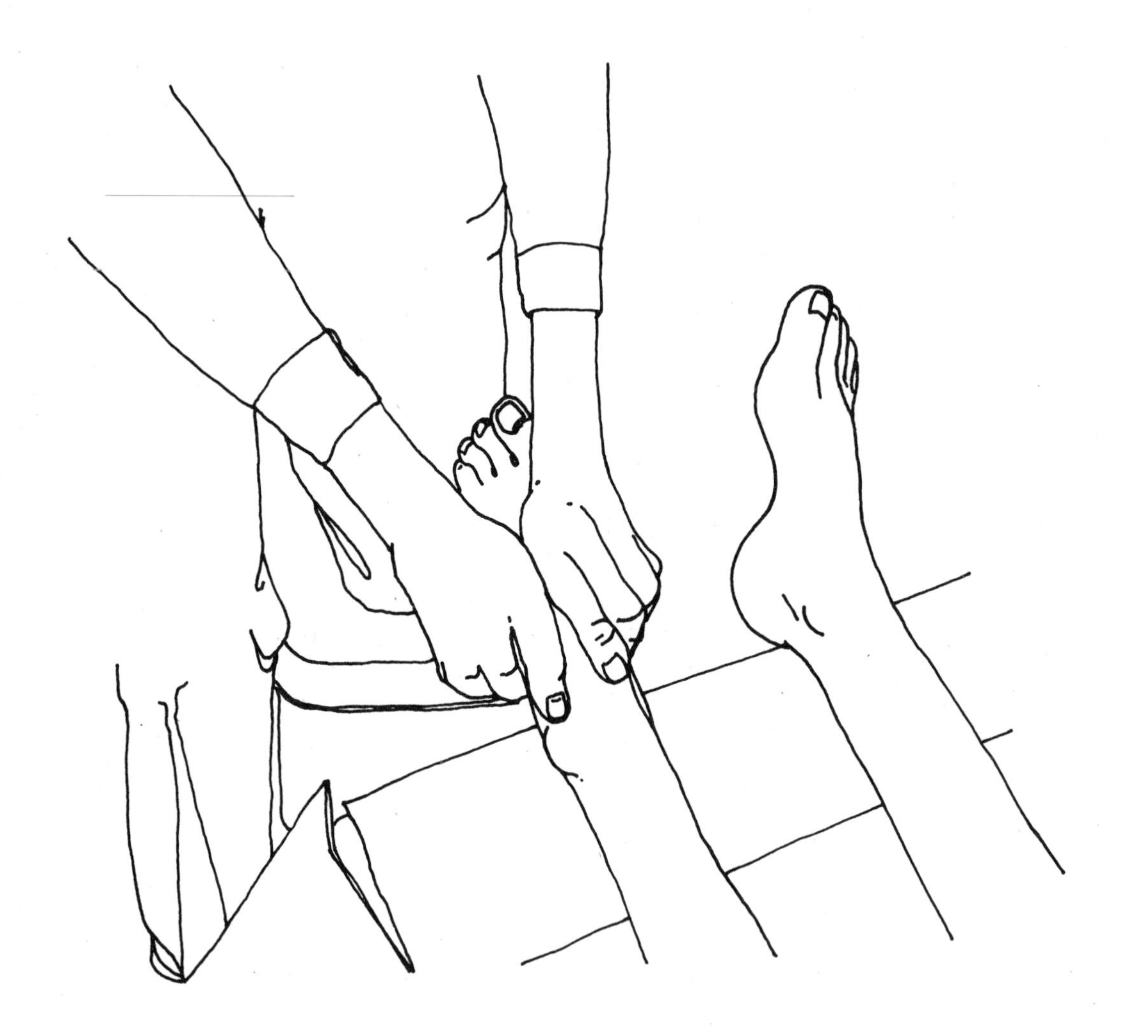

FOOT PRESSURE GLIDE

Grasp the leg above the ankle with both hands, thumbs on top and fingers on the bottom.

With a firm pressure, slowly glide your hands from the ankle, across the arch of the foot, ending at the tip of the toes. Curve your fingers around the bottom of the foot.

Start above the ankle again and repeat several times.

Do the other foot.

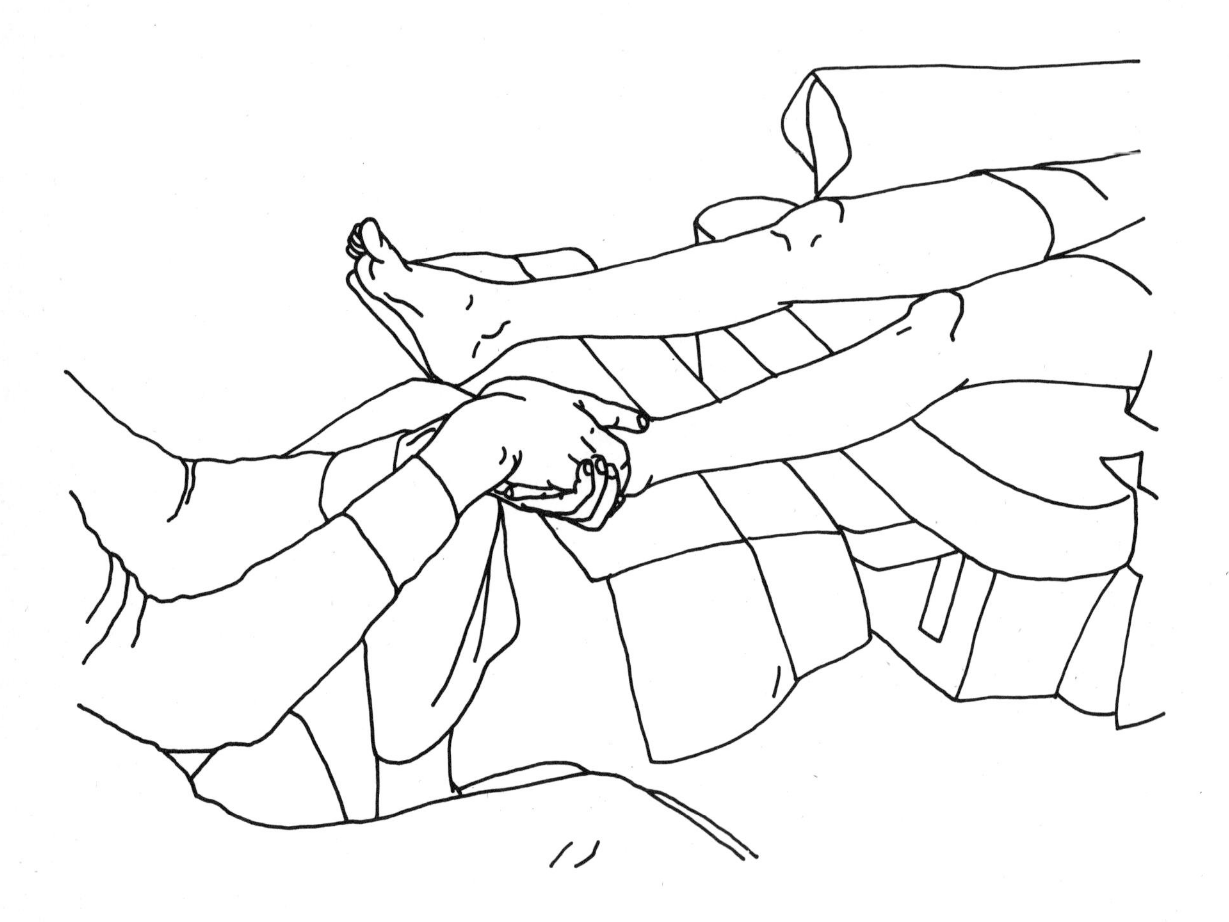

FOOT WARMING

Rub the palms of your hands briskly together until they feel pleasantly warm. Place one hand on top of the foot and one hand on the sole.

Switch top and bottom hands to get a slightly different feel.

Hold each foot with a firm, comforting pressure for at least 1 minute.

End the foot movements by rubbing a moisturizing cream or lotion over the top, bottom and between the toes of each foot. This feels exceptionally good.

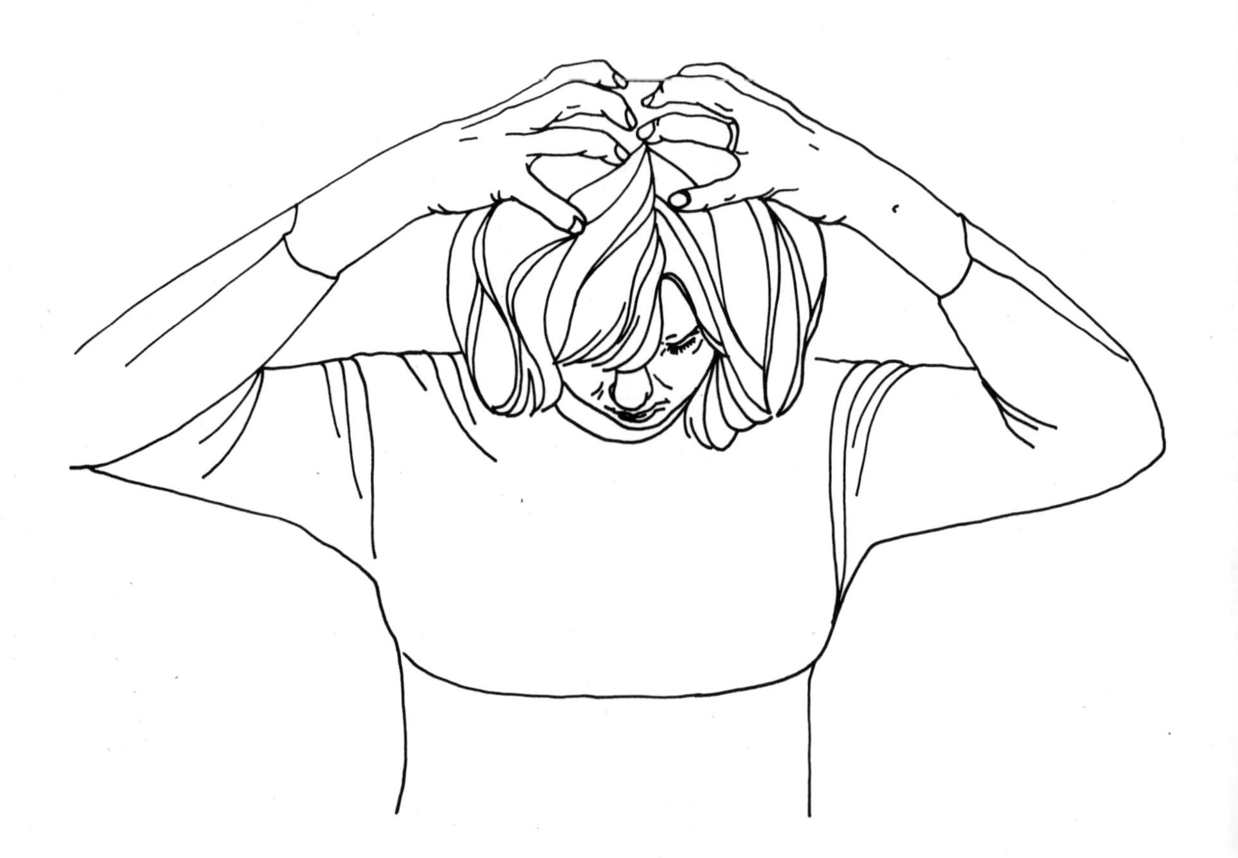

8

QUICK SELF-MASSAGE

It's always nice to relax completely while someone else gives you a soothing mini-massage. However, many times you're alone or no one is interested in working on you. When this happens you can always give yourself a massage. Care must be taken so that the muscle tension produced in your arms, back and shoulders while giving yourself a massage doesn't outweigh its benefits.

You can, however, work on certain parts of your body with positive benefits and a minimum of self-induced muscle tension. These include your scalp, face, back of the neck, midsection, lower legs and feet. In less than 10 minutes it's possible to give yourself a quick massage and still get good results. You don't need a massage table to do the movements, just use the floor, bed or couch.

SELF-MASSAGE MOVEMENTS

SCALP

Place your thumbs behind your head, and with fingers spread apart, slowly massage all over your scalp. Move your hands as necessary to reach the entire head area. Use enough pressure to feel the skin slide over the scalp.

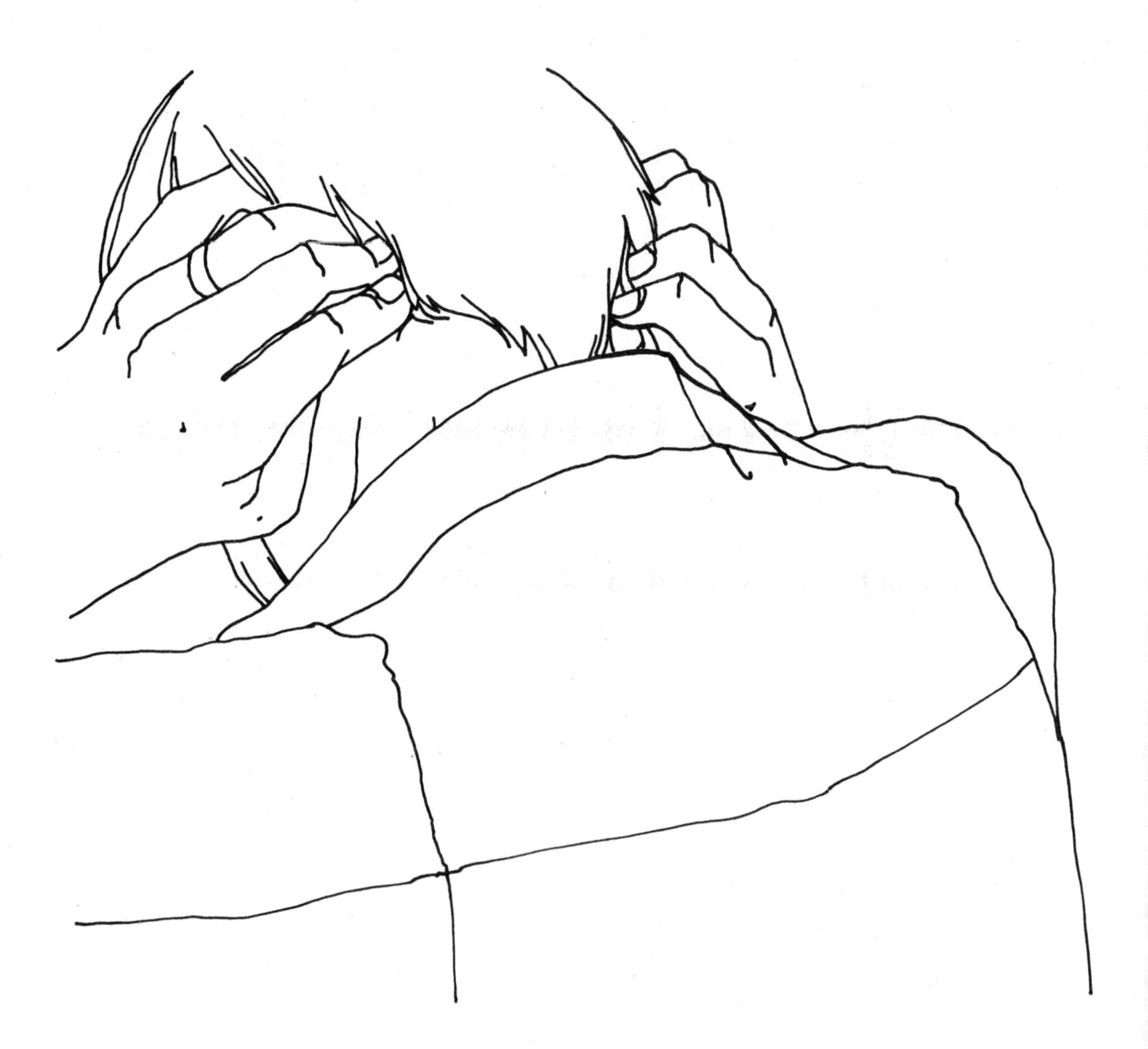

FACE

Use any of the face movements in Chapter 3—Forehead, Between Eyes, Temples, Around Eyes, Behind Ears and Jaw. You may find it more comfortable and easier to use your fingers rather than thumbs on the forehead. Also it may be easier to use your thumbs when stroking from the chin to the tip of the jaw.

EYE-CUPPING

As a final facial relaxer briskly rub the palms of your hands together until they feel good and warm. If you're wearing glasses, take them off. Contacts may be left in. Now, quickly cup your hands and place one over each eye. Cup your hands so that no light or outside air gets in. The palms should not touch your closed eyelids. Keep your hands in place for 15–30 seconds. Support your head in your hands and let your mind go blank.

Repeat if your eyes are extra dry or tired. You may want to put a couple of cleansing eyedrops in each eye before or after the eye cupping.

NECK

Place the first two fingertips of each hand in the notch where your neck meets the back ridge of the skull. Massage with a rhythmic, pulsating pressure for up to 3 minutes.

Use firm, steady pressure for 15 seconds and release for a few seconds, repeating for up to 3 minutes. (This is like the Trepidation movement, page 47.)

As an added movement, use the same fingertips to make small circles up and down your neck, working on the back and sides of the neck.

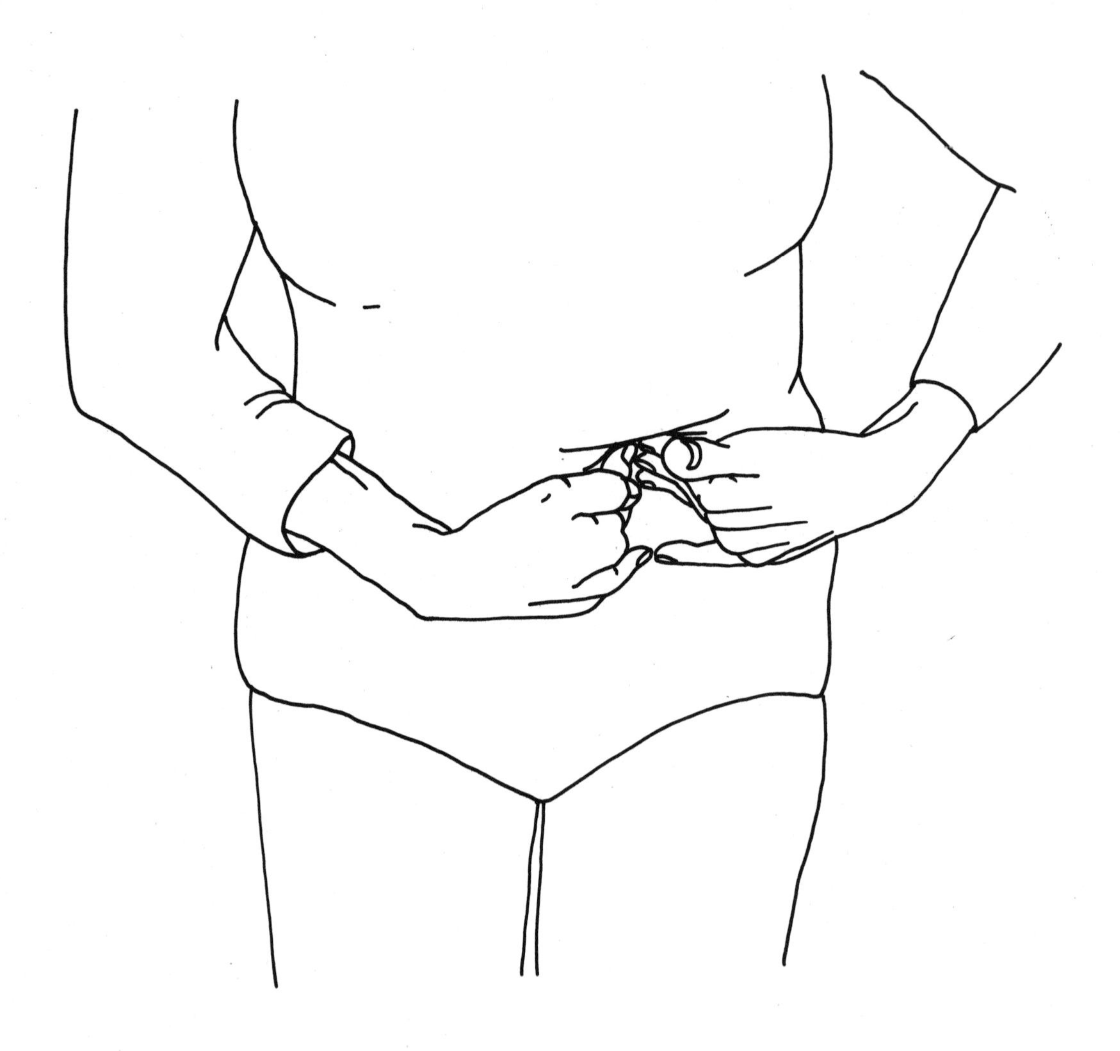

MIDSECTION

Constipation is a problem you generally don't want to discuss with others. You can help relieve your own constipation with a quick mini-massage to the intestinal area.

Lie down on your back and elevate your knees with your feet flat on the bed or floor.

Place the pads of the first three fingers of each hand on the right side of your intestinal area. Use firm pressure, and move slowly in small circles around the path of the colon. The colon runs up the right side, follows around and near the lower rib cage and down the left side toward the center of the pubic bone.

Always work from the right to the left side as this is the path that digested food takes as it moves through the colon. This is similar to the Colon (small circles) movement, page 89.

If constipation becomes a stubborn problem, spend extra time working on the left side. This is where the food waste tends to dry out and become hard and compacted.

Caution: Do not massage the intestinal area if pain is present as it may be due to appendicitis or other serious medical problems. Check with your doctor or health-care specialist if intense pain is present.

If you're frequently bothered with constipation, you can do a couple of simple things that will help you to regain a regular bowel schedule. The first thing to do to help matters along is to drink a large glass of water right after getting up in the morning. This helps the intestines move the previously digested food through the intestinal tract. If you can't take water first thing in the morning, then increase the amount of liquid you drink throughout the day.

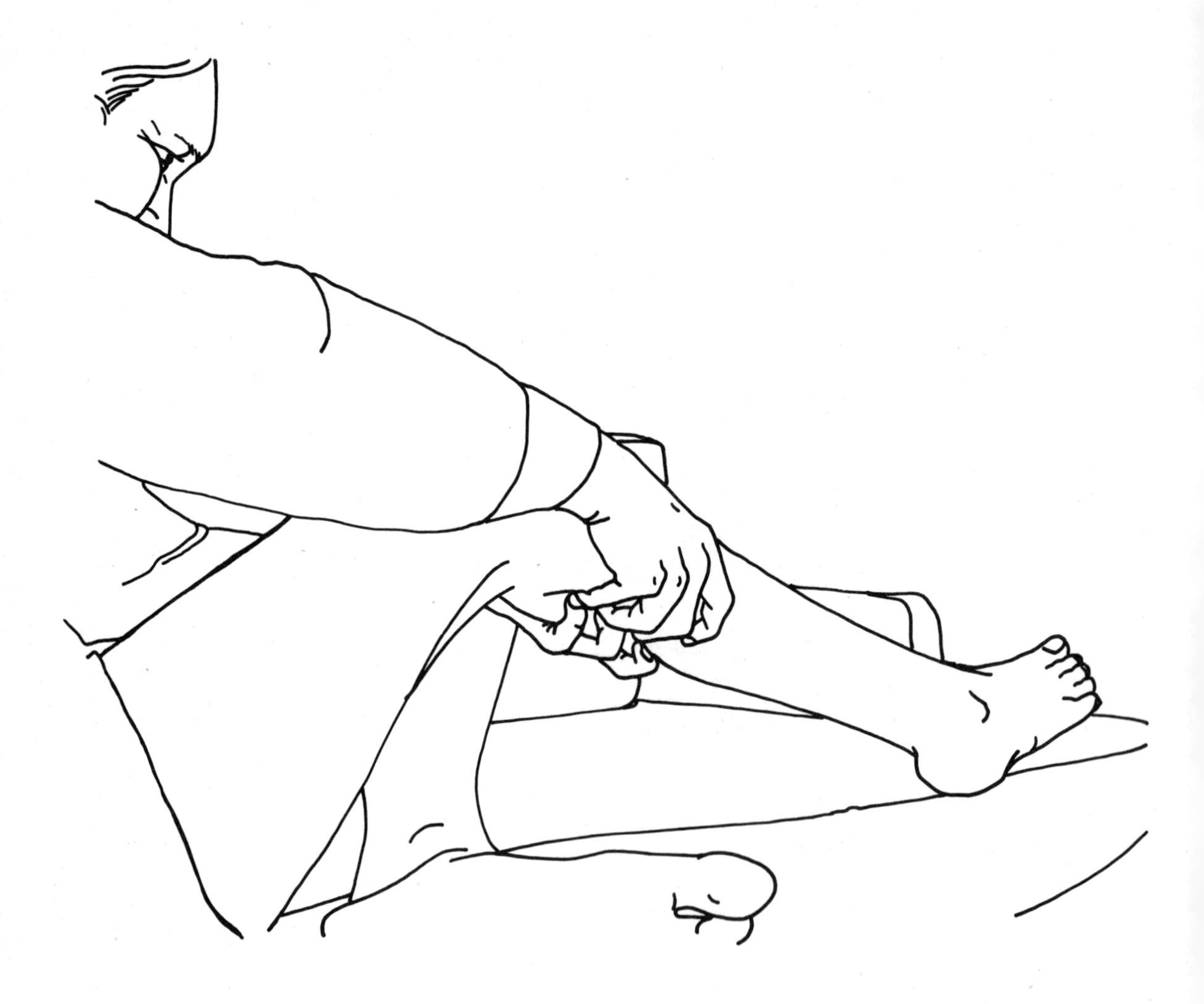

The second thing you can do is to breathe deeply, filling your lungs to their full capacity. As you breathe in, push your navel out as far as possible, and as you breathe out, pull your navel in as far as you can. Force your whole midsection to move in and out in an exaggerated manner. Do this forced push-pull movement ten to fifteen times at various points during the day. In addition, do the colon self-massage circular movements for a few minutes just before going to sleep and before getting up the next day.

You can use any of the movements in Chapter 6 to help relieve tension or cramps in the stomach and midsection.

CALVES

If you are sitting, place your foot on a footstool with your knee elevated. Place both of your hands around the calf with thumbs in the back. Knead the calf muscle between your fingers and thumbs.

If you are standing, place your foot on a low stool or chair. This time your fingers should be behind the calf. Again, knead the calf muscle between the fingers and thumb. Either position works. It just depends on what is most comfortable for you.

Use medium to heavy pressure to knead up and down the length of the calf muscle several times. Then switch legs.

You can also use the pads of the first three fingers of both hands to rub around and just behind the ankle bone. Make several circles in one direction and then reverse direction.

Sports trainers suggest you elevate your legs above the rest of your body to help remove the lactic acid in the muscles. When you're at home you can put your legs up on an ottoman, chair, couch, against the wall or anything else that's handy. Leave them there for 5–10 minutes.

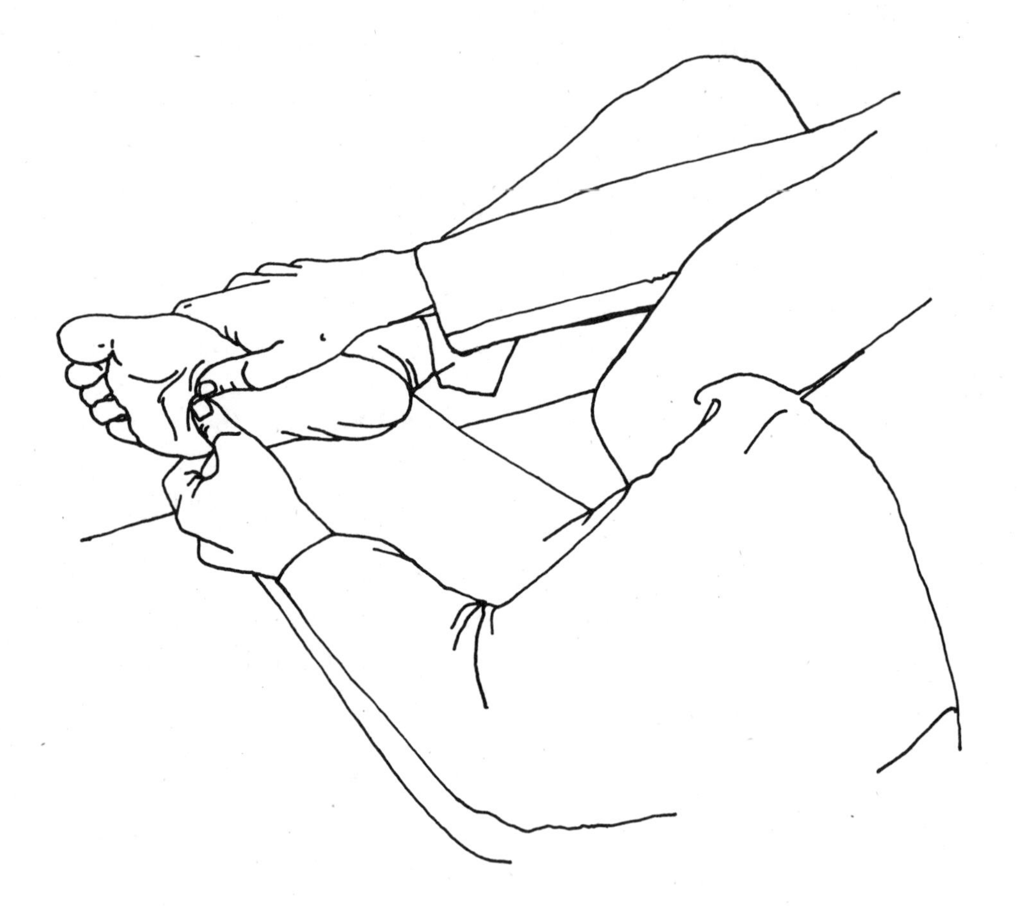

FEET

Sit on a chair or sofa, the floor or the edge of a bed to work on your feet. Bend your leg and bring your foot up so that you can reach and work on it comfortably.

Place the pads of both thumbs on the sole of your foot. Using firm pressure, massage from the base of your toes to your heel. Go over the entire sole several times. Then change to the other foot. You can also use your knuckles to massage the soles of your feet. In addition, rub each toe between thumb and forefinger with a slight pulling, twisting motion.

To give yourself a soothing footbath, add some Epsom salts to warm water and soak your feet for 15 minutes. Epsom salt is made up of tiny magnesium sulfate crystals. Magnesium is a good muscle relaxant, and when dissolved in water, it is readily absorbed by the tissues and its action helps to soothe tired, achy muscles or sprains.

After you've briskly dried your feet with a heavy towel, rub them with a moisturizing cream or lotion. Put on a pair of light cotton socks to help keep the moisture in your feet. If the weather is cool, top these with a pair of warm socks or lined house slippers and give your feet and legs a much-deserved break.

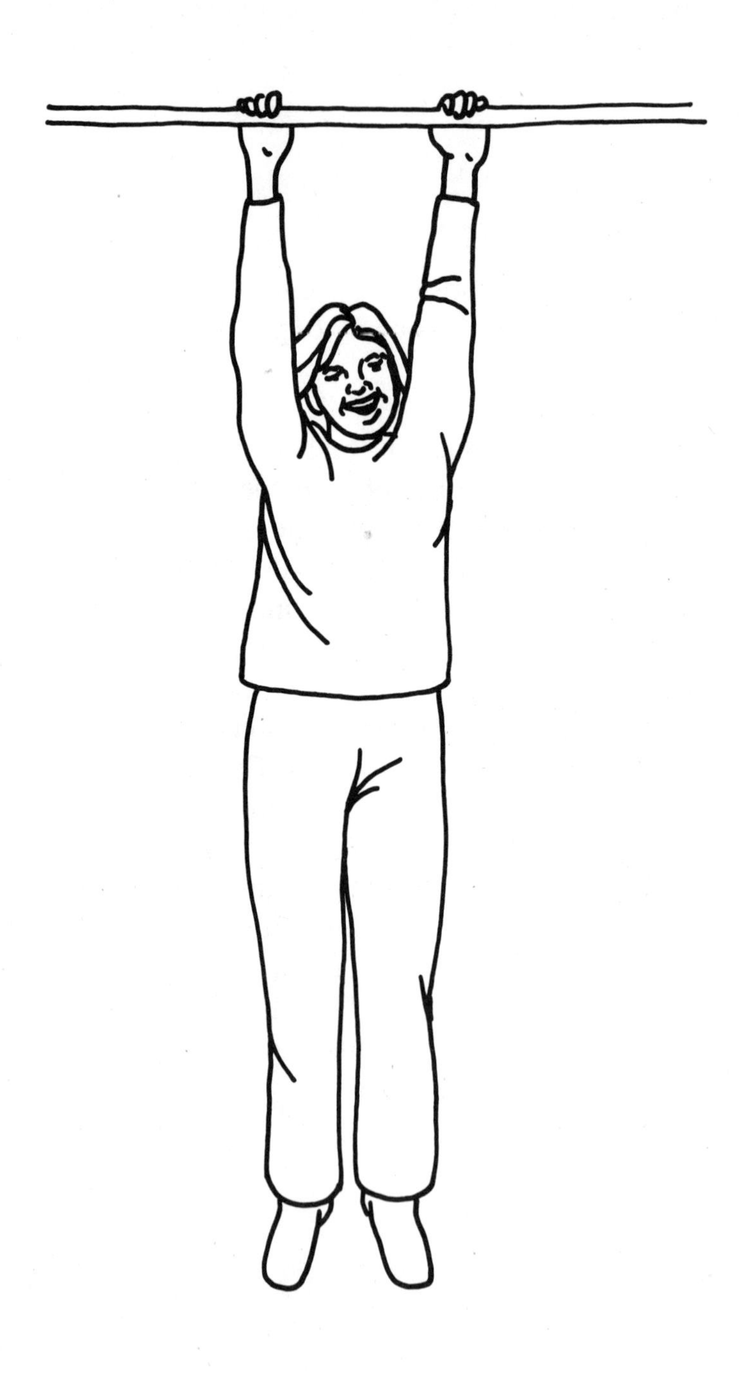

HANGING

Find a high bar or pipe that will support your weight. Grasp the bar firmly with both hands and bend your legs slightly so that your feet lift off the ground. Better yet find a bar or pipe high enough for you to hang straight without touching the ground.

Let the weight of your body stretch out the muscles in your shoulders and upper back. Hang until you've had a good stretch or until you just begin to feel uncomfortable.

Sturdy bars at various heights can sometimes be found in school yards or playgrounds at the park.

MASSAGE ACCESSORIES

A wide variety of massage accessories is available on the market today that can greatly increase the benefits of self-massage. They come in all shapes, sizes and styles. Pillows of various sizes with vibrators inside furnish self-massage to the neck, back, legs and feet. Some accessories only vibrate, while others provide both heat and vibration. One costly stuffed chair model vibrates, moves two rollers up and down your spine, furnishes heat on your back and plays stereo music, all at the same time.

Caution: All massage accessories or devices, whether mentioned in this book or not, should be used according to the manufacturer's directions. Don't use any of the electrical devices near water or when bathing. With any of these devices, overuse may result in sore muscles or injury. The safest approach is to use any of the accessories for a short period to begin with and gradually increase the time until you find optimal relief.

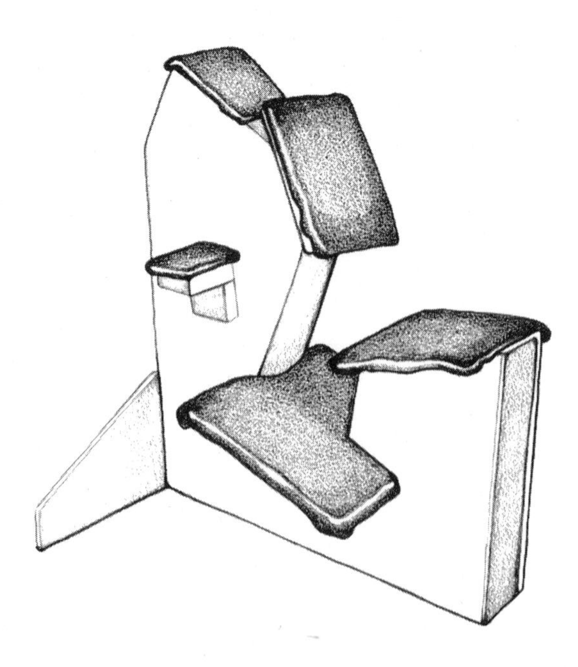

Massage Tables and Chairs

Although you don't need a massage table or massage chair to give a mini-massage or even a full-body massage, they make your job easier, especially if you give massages regularly. There's a big difference between giving a massage while standing at a massage table and giving one while sitting or kneeling on the floor. Your shoulders, back and knees tend to tire quickly when working from the floor. I recommend that you try working on the floor and then on any kind of table on which the person you're massaging will fit. If the table is too wide, have the person lie near the edge, and work on that side; then have her reverse positions so her other side is near the edge of the table. Assess the difference between working at a table and on the floor, and then decide if you want to buy a massage table or build a low-cost one of your own.

In the past, massages were given on the floor, a bed or a massage table. Now there is the newly designed massage chair for doing body work. The person receiving the massage sits in the chair leaning forward with his chest resting on a movable pad, the head resting on a padded headrest and the arms on padded armrests. The person may remain clothed or take his shirt off. The angled position of the receiver makes it easier for the giver to work without back strain. The massage chair offers a comfortable, relaxed position for both giver and receiver while providing easy access to receiver's head, neck, shoulders and back.

Massage tables and specially designed massage chairs are available from many sources. You can find out where to buy one if you contact a massage therapist in your area, pick up a copy of *Massage* magazine, or write to *Massage* magazine, P.O. Box 1389, Kailua-Kona, HI 96745.

If you want to make a massage table quickly and easily, for about $50, buy an 80 × 28 inch unfinished door blank and a pair of folding sawhorses at your local lumberyard or discount home center. Place the door blank on the sawhorses, put a foam pad or blanket on the door and, presto, you have an inexpensive massage table that can be easily stored away when not in use.

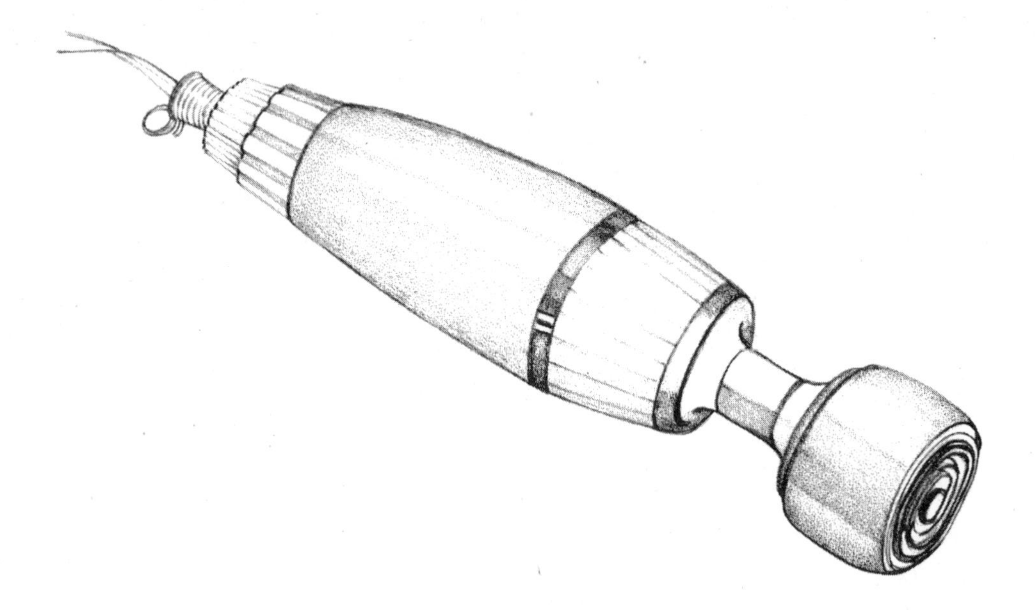

General Purpose Vibrators

Hand-held general purpose vibrators come in many shapes and sizes. They range in price from about $20 to $70. The smaller vibrators sometimes come with soft rubber attachments for use on skin, harder plastic attachments for deep muscle vibration, and even an attachment with rubber "teeth" for use on your scalp. Some vibrators have ridges or bumps on the vibrating head. Others use a curved plastic surface on the end of the head for directing deeper vibrating action into the inner muscle tissue. The illustration above shows one of the elongated models with a variable speed control at the cord end of it. The side of the head is made of rubber and the end is made of a firm, curved plastic.

Another type of hand-held vibrator has a small motor on one side and small flexible springs on the other. Your hand fits between the motor and the springs. The motor rests against the back of your hand, causing your whole hand to vibrate. The springs serve to hold the vibrator in place. You can direct the vibration through your fingers to the area you're working on. This type of vibrator is fine for massaging the scalp and shoulders.

Heavy-duty Vibrators

Heavy-duty vibrators cost about $100 and are usually lighter than they look. They're mainly designed for use on another person's back although they can be used, to a limited extent, on the legs, feet and top of shoulders during a self-massage. One model has a padded curved head which lends itself to use on the calves or thighs. Since the heavy-duty unit delivers a very strong vibrating action, it's recommended that you use it for only short periods of time on any specific part of your own or another person's body.

Super heavy-duty professional models are made in the United States and France for use by chiropractors, osteopaths, physical therapists and massage therapists. These furnish very deep, powerful muscle vibration and give more action per minute than any other units on the market. They also cost several hundred dollars and have a large assortment of attachments available. Never use any of the professional vibrators for more than a few minutes during any given mini-massage, because of their strong vibrating action.

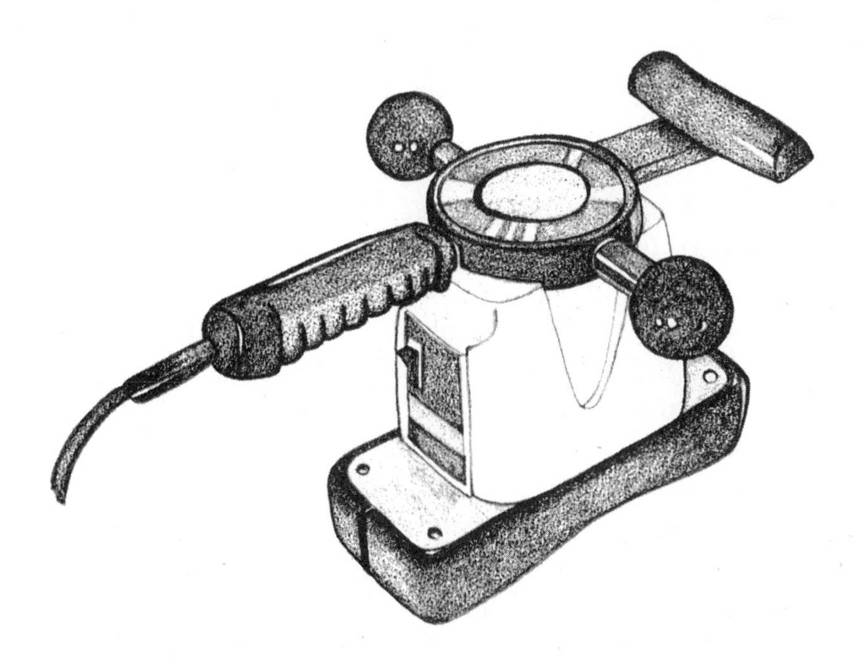

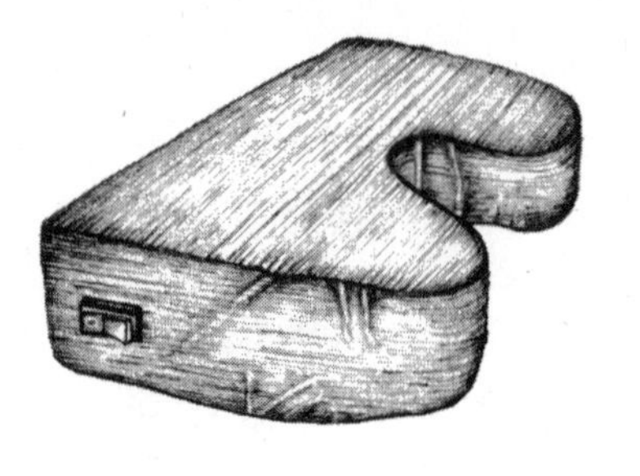

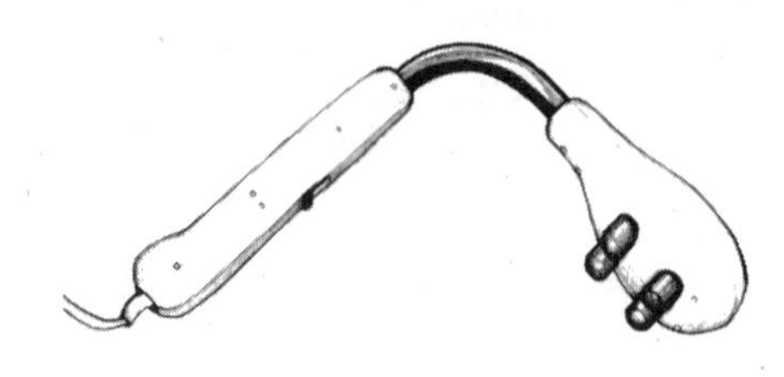

Special Purpose Vibrators

The illustration above (left) shows a pillow that's designed for use on the back of your neck. It's covered with corduroy and is turned on or off with a rocker-type switch on the side of the unit. While it does a good job on the neck, it doesn't do much for the upper shoulders unless someone pushes down on the pillow while it's vibrating. Sitting in a high-backed recliner seems to work best when using the neck vibrator as only part of the weight of the head and neck then rests on the pillow, allowing it to vibrate freely, as opposed to the full weight of the upper part of the body, which would come to bear on the pillow if you were lying down.

Self-actuated pillows have a built-in pressure-sensitive switch that starts the vibrating action when contact is made with the pillow. Take your weight off the pillow, and it stops vibrating. Place one of these behind your back, and lean against it while sitting on a chair, couch, car seat, or on the floor, with your back against a wall. When lying down, stuff one under your legs to relieve tired, sore calves. You can even sit in a chair and put your feet on the pillow, and it serves as a foot vibrator.

You can also make your whole bed vibrate. Some motels and hotels have units that cause the whole bed to vibrate for 15–20 minutes when you put a quarter in a metal box. Usually there's an address on the coin box where you can order a home unit for mounting to the underside of your bed. This type of vibrating bed is very relaxing after a long drive or a hard day's work.

Smaller battery-operated vibrator pads are available in a variety of sizes. Because of their size, they're handy for travel or work as well as at home. They fit easily into a shoulder bag, briefcase, suitcase, or the glove compartment of a car. They're suited for either self-massage or use on another person. These pads are also self-actuated and start when pressure is applied to the unit. You can hold one in your hand and press it against your body or place it behind your back.

There's even one model for use in your car. The folding seat and back cushion provide a vibrating massage when the cord is plugged into the cigarette lighter.

One special vibrator that's extremely well suited for a self-massage of the shoulders and upper back has an L-shaped handle and four fingerlike plastic nodes on the vibrating head which stimulate sore muscles. By holding it over your shoulder, you can reach the shoulder and mid to upper back. By positioning it at your side and letting the vibrating head reach around your back, you can reach all of your lower back. You can also use it to massage the buttocks and underside of your legs. It has two speeds: low, for a gentle massage, and high, for a deep massage.

In the Kamuela Museum located in the town of Waimea, on the big island of Hawaii, there's a "massage stick" that was used by royalty in the latter part of the 1800s for giving themselves a back self-massage. The servants of the royal family chose the tree branch used to make this stick with great care. It had to be a curved L-shaped branch with a small knot at the bottom of the lower stroke of the L. The special knot served as a kind of thumb pad. Strangely enough, the one in the museum really looks like a thumb pad.

Another totally different type of massager makes use of a Velcro fastener sewn to a wide band that fits around your waist, arm or leg. A small, electrical vibrator clips to the band over the spot you want massaged. When turned on, it massages the whole area around and under the band. One model comes with both a heat and a cold mode.

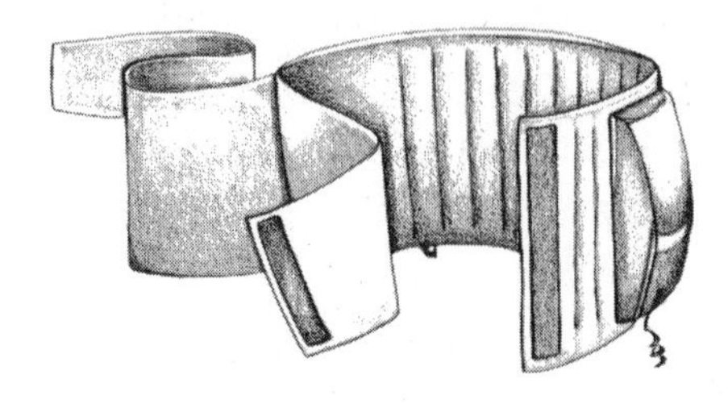

Foot Massagers

Feet get special emphasis when it comes to the variety of massage accessories available. There are several kinds of wooden devices available for self-massage of the feet. The top illustration on the facing page shows one made of cherry wood, with grooves of various sizes. It has rubber rings on both ends to help keep it from moving sideways. You place this device on the floor, put your bare foot on it and roll it back and forth. This is best if done when sitting, as you shouldn't put all your weight on the massager. Other models have wooden rollers or wheels on them. Although this kind of device is an inexpensive novelty of sorts, you may find some relief or pleasure in using one.

An editor in New York rolls her foot over a squash ball to give herself a quick foot massage. If you want to try something unusual, you can fill two high-top athletic or tube socks with enough dry soybeans to cover the sole of the socks. Put the socks on and stand up or walk around for a few minutes. Since the soybeans are small and hard, they get into all the critical areas on the bottoms of the feet and give them a quick foot reflexology treatment. Just don't try entering any marathon races or beauty contests while you're doing it.

There are also many electric foot massage devices available. The first category includes those that vibrate only. One foot massager is built as a unit with curved plastic vibrating heads mounted on top. You move your feet freely over the heads.

Another design (see middle illustration on the facing page) has a separate vinyl-covered slipper for each foot. The slipper-like pouch is open at the heel so that the foot can be easily slipped in or out. You won't have to sit around with your feet in one position—the slippers are attached by a strap so you can move each one separately. You have a choice of three vibration speeds, each with or without heat.

The bottom illustration on the facing page shows a deluxe footbath for soothing your tired feet. This model warms the water and has a built-in exerciser to massage your feet.

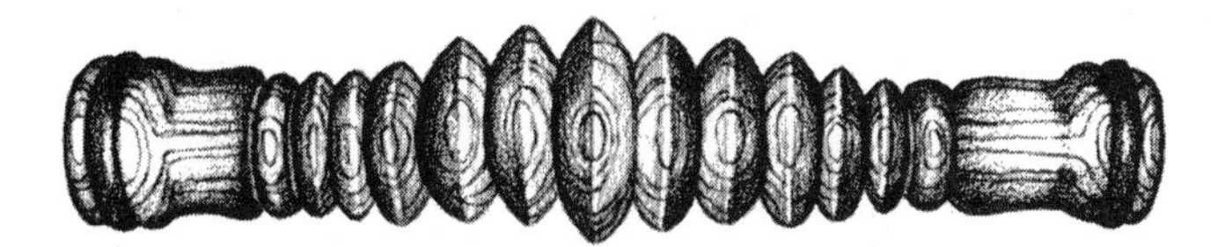

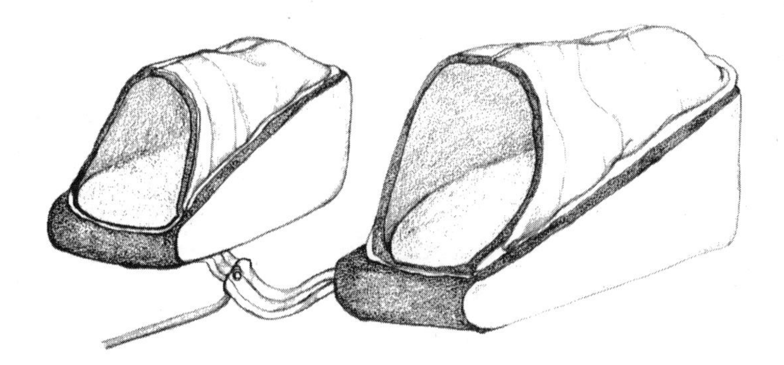

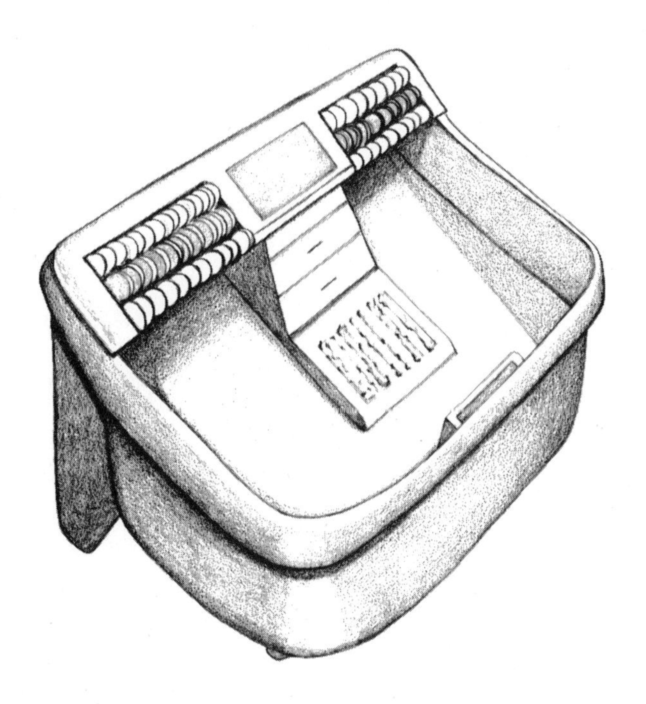

Heating Pads/Vibrators

Heating pads have long been used as a cure for tired, sore muscles. Many women find they provide relief from menstrual cramps.

The standard electric heating pad has a set of heating wires enclosed in a vinyl pad which is covered by flannel or another type of thick cloth. The heat control is mounted on the electrical cord. Heating pads provide dry heat, and some new models can be used to apply moist heat.

As previously mentioned, some back massagers provide heat as well as vibration. One model (see illustration below) has an adjustable pad that can be moved to various positions. Velcro strips mounted on the back of the vinyl heating pad hold the vibrator in place. The unit fits in a chair and is used for relieving tension in your back and shoulders. Placed under the legs, in bed or on the floor, it provides relaxation for tired or achy calves.

Caution: While using any heating pad, be careful that the unit doesn't become too hot and cause burns. You shouldn't use heat for more than 15 minutes at a time, and* never *go to sleep when using a heating unit.

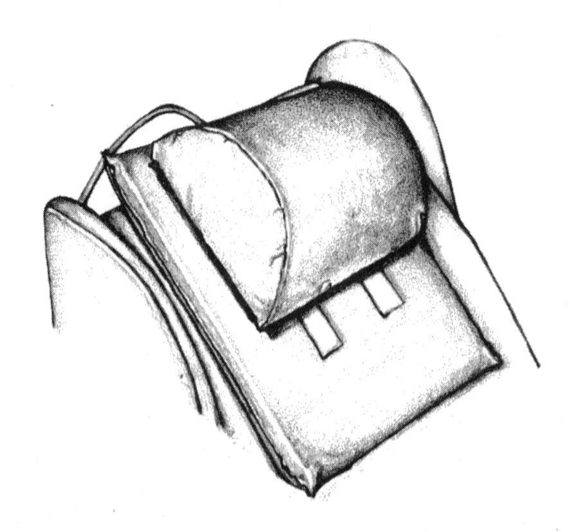

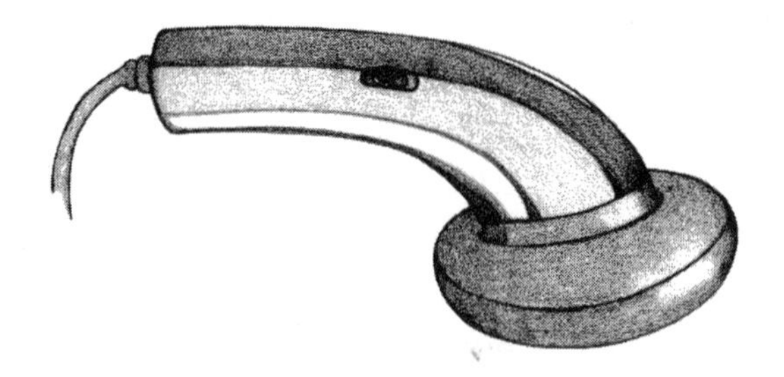

Heat Lamps

Heat lamps can be used to soothe sore and aching muscles before or after a self-massage or mini-massage. They come in many wattages and styles: there are floor lamp models and portable models that look like photographic back lights. The latter type clamps to the back of a chair or onto a shelf and swivels around to the proper angle and height. Be sure the portable lamp is secure so there's no danger of it falling and touching the exposed skin. Heat lamps should only be used for short periods of time and need to be adjusted so that the skin doesn't get too hot.

One type of heat lamp (see illustration above) is hand-held, and uses only 8 watts. It furnishes infrared shortwave light to relieve minor pain, minor joint irritation, muscular pain, backaches and trigger point muscular spasms. Place the heat lamp directly over or near the painful area. Sometimes the painful area isn't the source of the pain, so you may have to probe other spots to get the best results. You can hold the heat lamp in one spot or move it around the painful area. It's designed for use with the skin bare or through clothing, although with heavier clothing the heat takes longer to penetrate. Cream or oil may be used with the hand-held lamp if a cloth or paper towel is placed between the heat lamp and the bare skin. Treatments usually last from 5–15 minutes.

Caution: Heat lamps should not be used on varicose veins or in the abdominal region when pain is present. And,* never *let unattended children use one.

Hundreds of years ago, Hippocrates applied heat to wounds to speed up healing. This method is again being applied in hospitals today. Dr. Hunt and Dr. Rabin of the University of California, San Francisco, discovered in a study of hospitalized patients that when heat was applied to a wound, blood flow to the wound went up an average of three times over the normal rate. Oxygen content increased, which assisted in the healing process and in clearing bacteria away from the wound. Check with your doctor, health-care specialist or massage therapist if you have any questions about the use of any heat or massage device for treating a given disorder.

Muscle Stimulators

A muscle stimulator can help to break up muscle tension or to reduce the intensity of muscle spasms. The illustration below shows one type of accessory used to stimulate muscles so that they contract and release rhythmically. The stimulator sends a small but harmless current through the two moistened sponge pads to the muscle area being worked on. It is powered by two D-cell batteries, and the amount of current is adjusted by a slide switch. Other types of muscle stimulators allow adjustment according to pulse rate and intensity; some have a timer and manual or automatic polarity reversal. They range in price from $100 to $300.

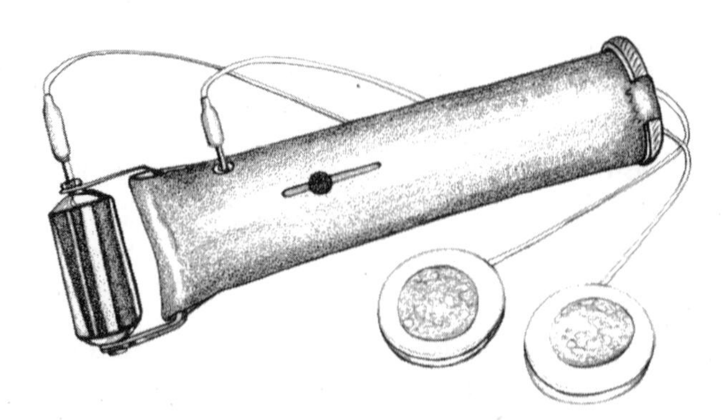

Ice Packs

Ice packs are about as old as the discovery of ice itself. They are used to reduce swelling in twisted or injured joints, to ease the pain of a toothache, to soothe a hangover and to relieve a nagging headache. There is no need to fumble with the old-style messy ice bag anymore. Reusable Blue Ice aid and ice packs are now available in many sizes and shapes and can be purchased at most drugstores.

Some ice packs are kept in the freezer for ready use. If the ice pack is frozen, place a damp cloth between it and your skin to prevent frostbite. Others are kept at room temperature, and by twisting the plastic bag, a substance is released that causes the temperature of the blue liquid in the bag to drop to near freezing. The bag is immediately placed on the site of injury.

If you're away from home, it's a good idea to carry an instant ice pack in your car or sports bag. Place the pack over an injury as soon as possible to relieve the swelling.

You can buy a special Blue Ice pack that's designed for use on the face, with cutouts for the eyes. This pack can be used either chilled or warmed. Use it chilled to ease tension headaches, relieve hangovers, refresh the face or soothe tired, puffy eyes. Chill it by putting it in the freezer for 15 minutes, or as directed. Use it warmed to ease allergy discomforts, soothe sinus pain, or to relieve head colds and congested nasal passages. Warm it by soaking it in a pan of hot water for 5 minutes. Follow the maker's directions for preparation and use.

Baths and Showers

A warm bath or sauna helps to relax your muscles. A 10–15 minute soak in a tub full of warm water is a wonderful way to relax after work or at the end of a day. Fill the tub until you can lie immersed with just your head above the water. If your tub has a built-in or portable Jacuzzi, aeration or whirlpool unit, so much the better. These units cause thousands of bubbles to pass through the water every minute. The bubbles in turn bump into all parts of your body and provide a gentle, stimulating effect. Whirlpool baths have been used by sports trainers and physical therapists for decades to help treat muscle strains and injuries.

The advantage of a shower over a bath is obvious—it's so quick and easy to undress and pop under a shower, as opposed to waiting for the tub to fill. You have more instant control over the water temperature with a shower. Pulsating shower heads are specially designed to provide a soothing, massaging action to your neck, shoulders and back. If you have a movable hand-held shower head you can direct the spray to selected parts of your body. If your muscles are especially sore, it's good to alternate hot with cool water a few times when you're taking a shower. The cool cycle needs to be much shorter than the hot cycle. As mentioned in Chapter 4, this helps remove the lactic acid from your sore muscles.

Much has been written about bathing over the years. A bath or shower should be a time to completely relax. If you find bath accessories help you relax, then by all means go ahead and use them. Add scents, oils, rubber ducks, toy sailboats, soft music or candles to your bath routine. A relaxing bath or shower is an excellent way to prepare for, or to end, any kind of massage.

A brisk rubdown with a heavy towel after bathing helps stimulate the skin, removes dead skin, stimulates circulation and brings about a kind of balancing of energy throughout the body.

9

MUSCLE STRESS BUSTERS

STRESS BUSTERS

Whenever your body is under stress from fear, worry or anger it tries to arm itself against the perceived threat. The rate and depth of your breathing changes, your blood pressure rises, adrenaline pours into your bloodstream, and your muscles instinctively tense up. This sudden burst of fight or flight energy can reverberate long after the triggering event is over. It is important to build up resistance to stress and to break the stress cycle as early as possible to avoid the long-term physical and mental effects we discussed early on in this book. Ask yourself questions like, "What is going on in my life to make me overly tense?" and "Is there something that I need to change?" This will help you locate and work on your own stressful areas.

In my book, *Stress Busters: Bust the Stress Before It Busts You*, two close friends talk to each other about stress. They discuss learning how to recognize good and bad stress, how to break bad reactions to stress early in the cycle, and ways to check your stress level during the day. *Stress Busters* describes many physical, mental and emergency techniques for busting stress that you can use anytime the need arises. Typically, a person doesn't get sick until sometime after a period of high stress or crisis. This is why it's important to build up resistance to high stress and do whatever you can to reduce the stress reaction while it's happening.

In the previous chapters of *Mini-Massage*, the emphasis has been on how to break muscle tension in certain target areas by means of massage movements and the use of massage accessories. Chapter 9 deals with alternate ways to relieve stress and muscle tension. They should be used in conjunction with mini-massage.

MUSCLE STRESS

As we've said before, one of the most common signs of stress is tense or tight muscles in your target stress area. If you normally tighten up in the shoulders when you're under stress and you find tightness in that area, then it's very likely you're under some kind of stress. This is true whether or not you *know* what's causing the stress. Muscle stress busters help you to define the early signs of stress in your target area muscles and to take some action to stop any further buildup. Besides halting any stress increase, you need to know how to reduce the tension and how to soothe and relax your target area.

If a muscle is overworked or remains tense over a period of time, actual soreness in the muscle can result due to a buildup of lactic acid in the muscle tissue. You need to realize that this is another early-warning system telling you that something isn't right. This soreness may also come from a pulled muscle or from a blow to the muscle itself. Cramps or a charley horse in the muscles are other forms of muscle stress and can be caused by deficiencies of minerals such as calcium and magnesium. Supplements of these two minerals, combined into one tablet, can be taken for a short time. Do take them together as both are necessary to proper mineral balance in the muscles.

Sometimes if the muscles are in severe spasms, a higher ratio of magnesium to calcium is necessary. Also, if the cramps are the result of prolonged exercise, it may be necessary to take potassium in some form to replenish the loss. Consult with a health-care professional on the proper form and amounts to take.

Another common location of soreness is in the tendon or cartilage that acts as a link between a muscle and a bone. If you place too much strain on a tendon, it can tear and become inflamed. The Achilles tendon is a common site of injury for football players.

There are several ways you can tell if your muscles are overly tense. First close your eyes and picture the muscles in your target area, and ask yourself, "Do the muscles in my [shoulders and neck] feel tense?" Another way is to look into a mirror and note the expression on your face. The face often shows signs of stress. This is especially true of people whose target stress area is in the forehead. They wrinkle the skin on the forehead or furrow the skin of the brow just above the nose and between the eyes. People with tension in this area often have a lasting crease or deep lines in their forehead.

Sometimes you can place your hand on the area, such as the shoulders or legs, and feel the tightness. Muscle hardness isn't always a sign of stress. In athletes and body builders it may be a sign of increased muscle tone. Just keep asking yourself, regardless of your degree of muscle tone, "Do I feel tense in this area?" If you've been tense for a long time, it may take a few mini-massages on your target area before you can tell the difference between a normal relaxed muscle with good tone and an overly tense, stiff muscle.

Once you know how to recognize muscle stress, you need to take swift action to break the tension before it becomes locked in and fixed. A somewhat novel way of reducing tension in the shoulders and upper back is to "bong" away the tightness. "Bongers" can be purchased in health stores. They consist of two rubber balls attached to flexible steel shafts with wooden handles. Hold one in each hand and drum away on the shoulders and upper back. (See illustration on page 144.) The amount of impact can be adjusted to suit the wishes of the receiver. You can also use them on yourself, although not quite as effectively.

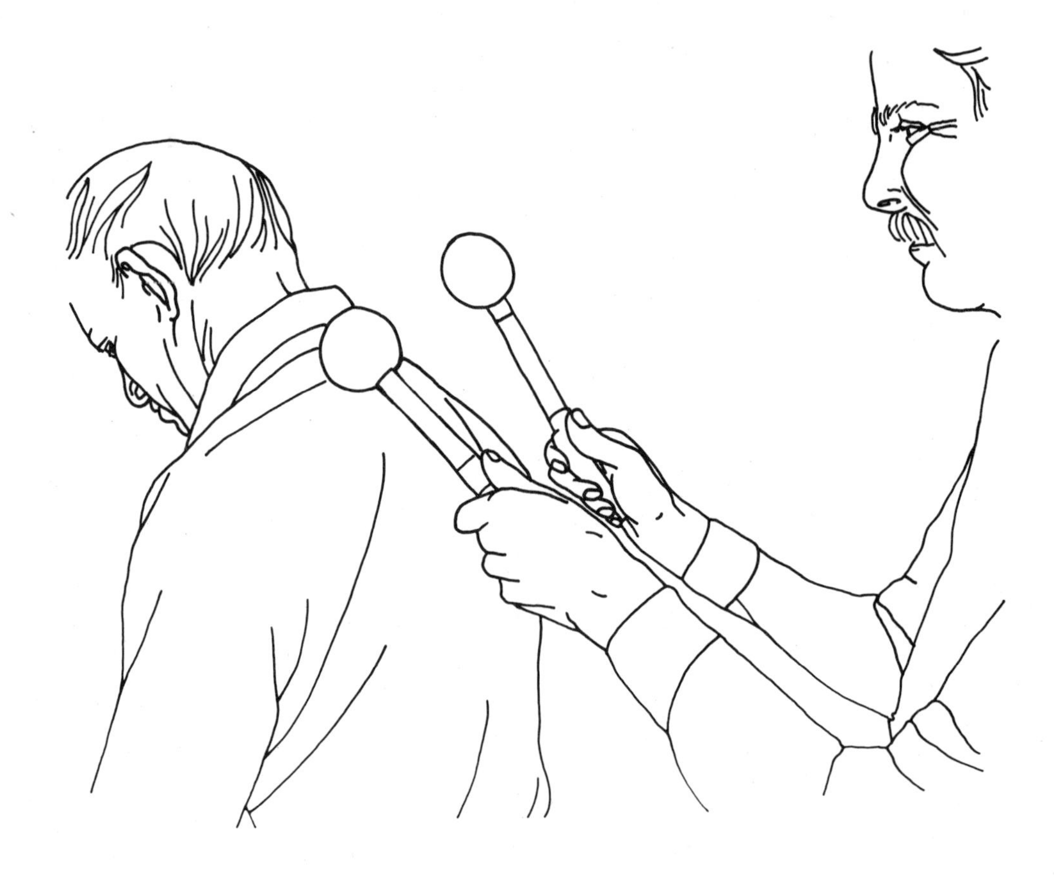

STRETCHING AND EXERCISING

It's a well-known fact that exercise helps reduce stress while building up energy and resistance to tension. Stretching and yoga exercises are especially good for relaxing tense muscles and keeping you limber. A daily exercise program will also enhance your overall sense of well-being. A shipping tycoon in Hong Kong takes an early morning swim in the cool waters of the bay every day. He says it helps him relax and meet the challenges of his complex, multibillion-dollar business.

One simple way to release tension in target area muscles is to exaggerate the tension. If, for example, you get tense in the shoulders and you want to break the tension, tighten and hunch your shoulders for 15 seconds—then release them all at once. After doing this several times you'll feel your shoulders becoming less tense.

Yawning also has a beneficial, relaxing effect. All animals, even ants, yawn. While you stretch, take a deep yawn, then let all your muscles relax at once.

There are many good books and programs on exercise, yoga and stretching. Choose one that suits your needs, likes and life habits.

INS AND OUTS OF BREATHING

Abnormal breathing is another sure sign of a stress reaction. Two kinds of irregular breathing occur in people under acute stress. Either they hold their breath and breathe so shallowly it's hard to tell whether they're breathing at all or they breathe so rapidly and deeply that they verge on hyperventilating. Heavy breathing due to physical exertion doesn't count. I'm referring to heavy breathing for no apparent physical reason.

Much has been written about how to breathe properly. Breathing is something that occurs involuntarily, although you can change its rhythm anytime you want to. Breathing exercises are many and varied. Some experts say to take a deep breath to a count of six, hold for a count four and exhale to a count of six. Others say to inhale for a count of eight, hold for a count of eight and exhale for a count of eight.

However you do it, the main thing is to bring your breathing back to a more normal rate if it's way out of line. Check your breathing during the day or when you feel you may be under stress. If it's either very shallow or very deep you need to bring it back to a more relaxed and stable pace. If you're among people, go someplace where you can be alone for a few minutes. If you're breathing shallowly and holding in your breath, take several deep breaths. Deep, full breathing will make your abdominal area move out while inhaling and cause it to fall back while exhaling. Don't think about counting or holding your breath. Just breathe deeply several times and exaggerate each inhalation and exhalation. The idea is to break the pattern of held-in, shallow breathing.

If you find you're breathing rapidly and deeply, sit down, close your eyes, and just let your body go limp until your breathing has slowed down. If you're hyperventilating, it's been recommended by health-care specialists that you breathe into a brown paper bag for a few minutes. The collection of carbon dioxide in the bag helps to slow down the rapid breathing. Don't put the bag over your head, of course.

LIGHTEN UP

When your muscles are tight, they're fighting—against the inertia of the rest of your body—to keep you relaxed and in balance. You need to loosen up and let go of this rigid body posture. There are several things you can do to help lighten up. When you're walking somewhere, don't hold your head down and look directly at the ground or sidewalk where you are walking. Keep your head up and focus your eyes on some point a short distance ahead of you. Walk with your shoulders erect but in a relaxed position. Notice how you walk when you're happy or excited. Your step is livelier and you seem to move about without any effort. Keep this in mind when you feel tense and try walking as though you were happy and excited.

Humor is a great way to lighten up. A good laugh helps you lighten up while lessening muscle tension. Laughter not only serves as good preventive medicine and a tension reliever, but it can help you recover from an illness. As a result of Norman Cousins' research and writings, the medical community, and patients in general, are now more aware of the helpful effects of laughter in the treatment of disease. Cousins undoubtedly agrees with Proverbs, 17:22, which says, "A merry heart doeth good like a medicine." When you laugh your brain releases a host of "positive" chemicals. These chemicals—endorphins—make you feel better and more relaxed, which in turn may help your body's natural healing powers to take over.

Try something fun and harmless to loosen up. Do something a little crazy. A publisher in Texas starts off each day by sounding an "uah-duh-duh-tah-tah-tah" football game-like charge on a kazoo. Immediately after, he fires a shot with his toy six-shooter cap pistol. That way, he says, "I start every day off with a charge and a bang!"

Silly, yes. Stupid, no. If it helps you to start the day on an upbeat note, and it's not irritating or harmful to another person, then go ahead and do it. Sometimes the sillier, the better the effects. A bank executive in St. Louis says she sings everything from operatic arias to country music in the shower each morning. It helps her approach the serious business of the day on an up beat. A freeway commuter in Los Angeles makes absurd sounds when driving to and from work. The worse the traffic, the crazier the sounds. What works for discharging tension in one person, however, could have the opposite effect in someone else. So you need to custom design your own "crazies" and use them as you like.

One of the greatest performers in sports history, Greg Louganis, used his own brand of tension reliever during the 1984 Olympics. Before his last dive he was nervous because he knew he could be the first person ever to go over a perfect 700, and the earlier dives had gone exceptionally well. Greg knew from experience that tensing up or clutching at this point might blow the whole day. Even though he was in no danger of coming in second, he wanted this final dive to be as flawless as possible. In order to be calm and relaxed, he psyched himself up by singing, "I Believe in Myself" from the musical *The Wiz*. Greg won with 710.98 points—a previously unheard-of feat—more than 10 points over a perfect score. His record may never be broken. His special way of relaxing worked fine.

We live in both a very serious and a very playful universe. Anthropologists say the human form is slowly reshaping itself towards neoteny. Ashley Montagu, in his book *Growing Young*, talks a lot about neoteny. He says that the rate of maturation of the human species is slowing down so that adults are retaining more and more childlike features. The shape of the face and head is no longer the sloping Neanderthal look, but one that presents a softer more graceful appearance. Along with the change in physical features there is a tendency to more playfulness in the course of one's life. Being playful is a natural tendency which probably has biological usefulness in offsetting the serious and weighty side of life. As the old saying goes, "All work and no play makes Jackie a very dull person." Or to quote Tom Robbins, "It's never too late to have a happy childhood."

MINI-VACATIONS

Take a mini-vacation during the day. This may take the form of a few minutes spent thinking about a place you've been, a place you'd like to visit, someone you'd like to be with or something you'd like to do. It may involve going someplace new for lunch or visiting a favorite shop after work. Even during a work break you can let your mind roam to a place or situation far removed from your present circumstances.

Try doing something different on your break. If you work at a desk most of the day, instead of sitting down during your break, take a walk inside your building, or even go outside for a short walk if the weather's nice. If you normally stand up most of the day, take a load off your legs and feet, and sit down to read or chat with someone.

Another way of breaking up the day is to take a mini-vacation on the telephone. Call a friend and talk about something you both enjoy doing. Don't focus on problems. Keep the conversation on the light side. Let your thoughts "blue sky" for a while and stretch the limits of your imagination, even if they are little more than whimsical daydreams.

MUSIC

Music sparks all kinds of emotions. It's been used for centuries to please, excite and relax. With the number of recordings available, you'll find music to fit any kind of mood. Music helps break the boredom in fitness classes by injecting some spirit and rhythm into the exercise routine. It can also help you relax when driving, shopping, or working in the office or at home. Certain pieces will get your juices going and other tunes may lull you to sleep. Pick the kind of music you like to relax or unwind with, and play it when you're feeling tense.

I often use music to write by, depending upon the mood desired. If I'm feeling tired or sleepy, I'll play some hot guitar or lively jazz. If I'm feeling antsy, I'll play some mellow pop or light classical music.

GETTING QUIET

During the seventies, various forms of meditation were the in thing. You could consult a guru, take a meditation course, read a book or listen to a tape on how to meditate. Today, you can learn on your own to just sit quietly for a few minutes during each day. Getting quiet doesn't call for any special or strict training, and it costs you nothing. You merely allocate some time each day to sit and allow yourself to become quiet. You don't force anything. You don't need to repeat a word or phrase for it to be effective. All that's necessary is to sit comfortably for a few minutes or for as long as you like and let all your cares and troubles fade away. It may be hard at first, but the more you do it, the easier it gets. Don't worry about your chattering brain, or thought machine, it will learn to be quiet after a time. Remember, your brain needs to relax just as the muscles in your body need to relax.

TAKE A MUSCLE BREAK

Some Japanese corporations find that output goes up and morale is higher when employees take a 30-second muscle break every 20 minutes. They do a series of short muscle stress-busting exercises to relieve tension and refresh their spirits. These exercises are in addition to their regular morning and afternoon work breaks.

Here are three easy isometric exercises to relieve neck and shoulder tension by forcing one muscle group to work against another to produce contraction in the desired muscles.

Place the palm of your hand against the side of your head just above your ear (see opposite, top). While trying to push your head toward your shoulder, resist the pressure by pushing in with the palm of your hand. Hold for 5 seconds. Relax. Now switch sides, placing your other hand against the other side of your head.

Place both hands behind your head and interlock your fingers (see opposite, middle). While pushing back with your head, pull forward with your arms. Keep your elbows in front of you rather than straight out from your sides. Hold for 5 seconds. Relax.

Move your hands to your forehead, interlock your fingers, and while pushing forward with your head, pull back against your forehead (see opposite, bottom). Hold for 5 seconds. Relax. To help balance the muscles in your neck and upper shoulders, hunch and roll your shoulders for another 5 seconds. Then let your arms and shoulders hang limp for 5 seconds.

Other muscle stress busters you can do anytime include rotating your head slowly in full circles in one direction and then in the other direction. Stretch out your arms in front of you, then straight out from your sides, and then directly above your head. Swing your arms in full circles in one direction, then reverse the swing. Sit down, elevate your feet slightly and rotate them in each direction. Now, point your toes straight out as far as is comfortable and then bring them back toward your body, stretching the backs of your calves. Stand up and shake your body all over. And finally, as an energizer and re-

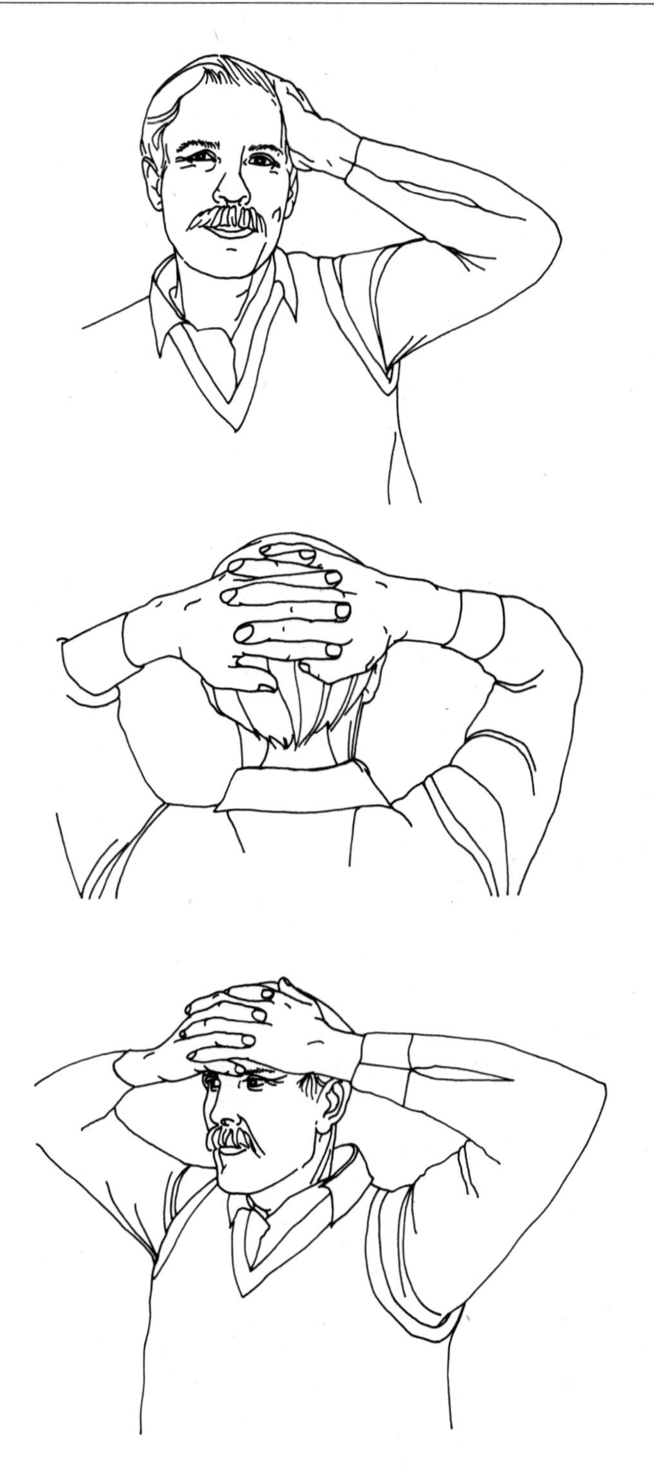

laxer, lightly slap or tap as much of your body as you can reach.

These simple tension relievers can be done almost anywhere and anytime. If you feel yourself getting tense during your daily routine, take a few minutes to stop and stretch the tension out.

THINKING ABOUT GOOD TIMES

Negative moods affect your body as well as your mind. They may cause your brain, adrenal glands and gallbladder to release harmful chemicals, and they can cause some of your muscles to tense up. If you find your thoughts are running wild on the negative side, switch to a good-times thought cycle.

Defuse the negative cycle with a sudden flurry of happy thoughts. A famous novelist uses the words, "CANCEL, CANCEL," when her thoughts start rampaging on the dark side. She immediately thinks about something she is looking forward to doing. She steps in quickly before the negative thought chain gathers extra energy.

POSITIVE REMINDERS

Positive reminders help brighten your day and relieve tension. You may have a special quote, poem, photograph, drawing, poster or letter that makes you feel good. If so, frame it and hang it on the wall at home or work. If a new word, phrase or quotation catches your attention, write it on a Post-it slip and stick it where you will see it during the day. Write yourself a positive reminder to take a stress break during your waking hours, whether you're at work, at home or traveling.

A photographer in Mexico enlarges a different photograph each month and mounts it on a bare wall in his living room. He says it helps to boost his spirit and keep his thoughts on the grandeur and mystery of life.

SLEEP

The position you sleep in has a great deal to do with how rested and relaxed your muscles are the next day. The recommended sleep positions are on your back or on your side. When you sleep on your back, your head should not be elevated too high. If you sleep on your side, keep your legs somewhat together—if you sleep with legs drawn up, draw up both legs, or if you sleep with legs stretched out, keep them both straight. If you're bothered by your knees knocking together place a small pillow between them. Sleeping with only one leg drawn up can put an unnatural twist on your spine. Keeping your legs together, in the same position, helps to avoid this twist. (See illustrations on following page.)

Sleep experts recommend that you not sleep on your stomach as this puts pressure on the muscles in your neck, shoulders and lower back. Of right-handed people who sleep on their stomachs, 85 to 90 percent will sleep with their heads to the left. Over a period of years this causes certain muscles in the neck to shorten while others lengthen, and it puts a strain on the cervical vertebrae. Also, as one leg is usually hiked up, a strain is put on the lower lumbar vertebrae. These unnatural twists put pressure on muscles in the back and on the spine itself, and may leave you feeling tense rather than rested.

WAKING UP

Get your muscles going by having a good stretch, from head to toes, before you get out of bed—like a cat does when it gets up from a nap. Have a healthy yawn with all the sound effects if you like. But don't push yourself too hard when you first get out of bed. Give your body a chance to adjust itself from the several hours of lying down to suddenly standing upright. You don't want to overdo it. Many heart attacks take place from about six to nine in the morning, so start your day gradually instead of rushing out of bed like someone fleeing from a fire.

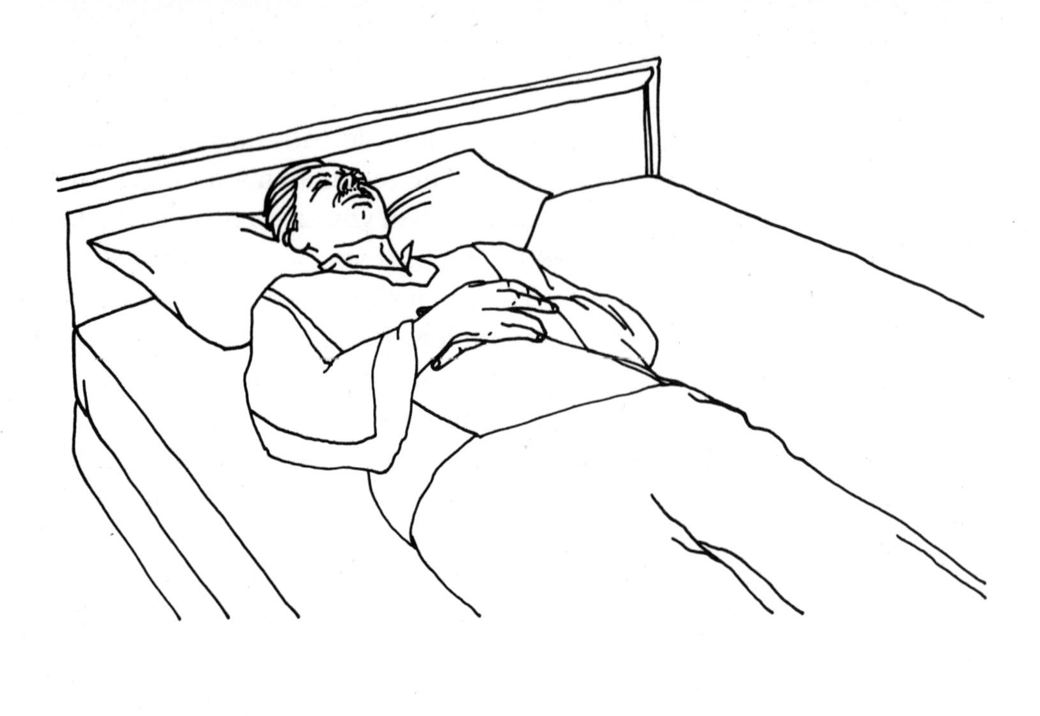

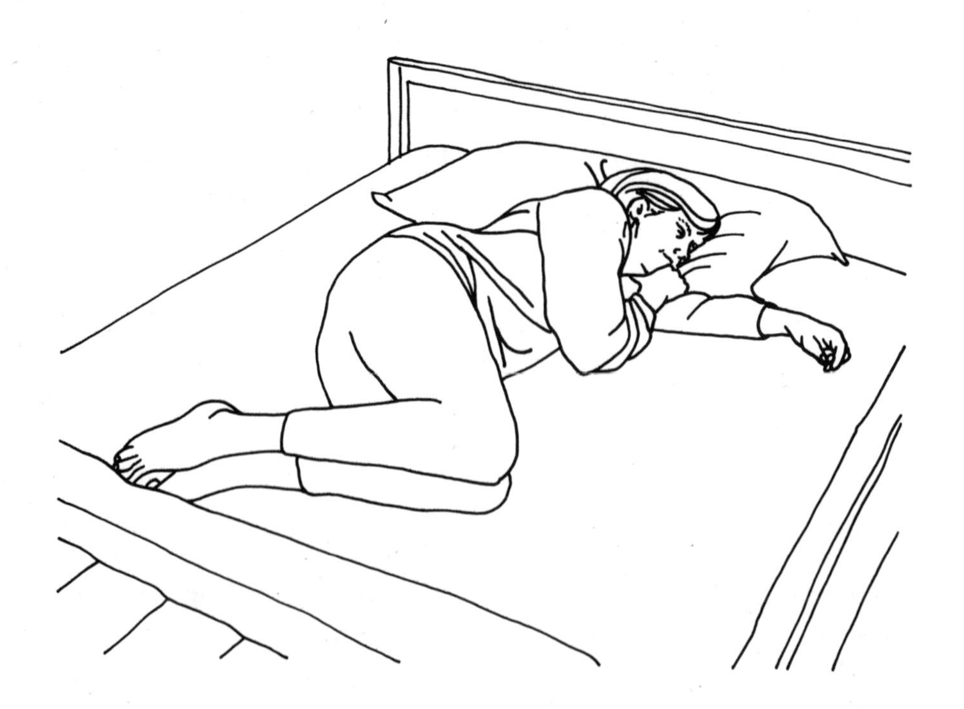

UNDERDO, NOT OVERDO

Avoid overexercising or overdoing any other form of physical activity, especially if pain is present. The tennis player who ignores pain in the shoulder or elbow may wind up with bursitis or "tennis elbow." Joggers or runners who insist on running even when their knees ache, their arches hurt or their shins are painful may soon not be able to run at all. These could be signs of a more serious problem, such as a torn tendon, a hairline fracture of the arch or a bad case of shin splints.

Of course, pains in the chest or the upper arms and shoulders should always be heeded as these could be warnings of an actual or impending heart attack.

Learn what mini-massage movements best help you or the person you're working on. Focus on these movements during any mini-massage. Throughout the day, use some of the muscle stress busters, or come up with some of your own.

LONG LIFE

The Committee for an Extended Lifespan, San Marcos, California, did a survey of 1,000 Americans who lived to be 100 years old or older. Each person's age had been documented by checking Social Security records.

The committee wanted to find out what physical or mental makeup or qualities these people had that enabled them to outlive the average American by 30 or more years. Members of the committee had certain preconceived notions about diet, personal habits, heredity and affluence, and how these might relate to long life. But none of these factors turned out to be crucial in assuring a lengthy lifespan. For example, many of the centenarians were poor, and had short-lived parents.

The committee did, however, find some basic patterns for long life. They found the centenarians did things in moderation. Three meals a day was the norm. Smokers either stuck to a couple of pipes or cigars daily, or they smoked cigarettes without inhaling. Those who drank alcoholic beverages did so sparingly. The habit to which longevity was most often attributed was going to bed early in the evening and getting up early in the morning. A large number were believers in a Divine purpose to life on earth. Many were self-employed and felt that hard work and keeping busy were important. The majority were self-sufficient, as much as was possible, and reported such things as "taking care of myself" and "never letting anything bother me" as major factors for a long life. Maybe a frequent mini-massage would have been one of the reasons cited had they known about its helpful effects in reducing stress.

In addition to the expected replies given above, the centenarians put forth several more unusual suggestions for long life:

1. Get plenty of rest. Sleep 10–12 hours per day.
2. Never sleep over 4 hours per day.
3. Sleep with your hat on.
4. Sleep with your feet pointed south so that magnetic vibrations from the north will pass through your body and out through your feet, ordering and harmonizing all systemic functions in the process.
5. Sleep with your feet pointed north so that magnetic vibrations from the north will pass upward to your brain with rejuvenating effects.
6. Abstain from meat, eating only raw fruits, vegetables and nuts.
7. Abstain from meat, eating only cooked fruits and vegetables.
8. Eat a pound of lean meat every day.
9. Get plenty of exercise.
10. Stand on your head for at least 5 minutes daily.
11. Shun physical activity. Conserve your energy.
12. Abstain from sex.
13. Have plenty of sexual activity.
14. Take steam baths.

15. Take lukewarm baths.
16. Take a cold shower every morning.
17. Bathe in ice water.
18. Never shock your system with cold water.
19. Get plenty of sunshine. It is the source of all energy and health.
20. Avoid sunlight. It causes cancer.
21. Don't cater to your appetites and whims. Observe strict self-discipline. Don't expect life to be too great, because it isn't. Prepare for the worst, and you'll never be disappointed.
22. Eat what you want, when you want it. Sleep when you're tired, and rise when you feel rested. Worry about nothing, think young—and have fun!

The committee concluded that maybe each thing works for somebody because that person believes in it. Or maybe the person would have done just as well without it. Maybe even better—who knows.

Each of us reacts to the world in a different way. What's stressful for you may cause little or no reaction in someone else. The opposite is also true: what helps you to relax and break the stress cycle may not work for another. Remember, what works for you is what counts! Whether you succeed in locating causes of stress, finding ways to relax, or developing personal methods to extend and improve your life, the final advice given by the Committee for an Extended Lifespan is something to mull over: "Take your choice from the list. Just don't try them all at once!"

INDEX